POPPING

ACNE

MYTHS

FOR SABINA

Making a journey in the dark, it's easy to get lost.

You are the light that guides me forward.

DEAR READER,

Acne is a tricky disease. Not only does it cause red, inflamed marks in the worst places possible, but it also has ramifications that run much deeper than our skin. When it's at its worse, our self-confidence takes a nosedive, and we become more depressed, anxious, and recluse. These disorders can persist long after the primary disease itself is treated. It's no wonder that the dermatology industry is worth billions of dollars today.

Acne can also be a frustrating disease to treat. We're constantly bombarded with misinformation about what causes this illness and "sure ways" to treat it. Common wisdom clashes with scientific knowledge often for acne. This is also part of the reason why I started this book. There are many misconceptions about what causes pimples and what you need to do to heal your skin. For anyone new to this topic, it can be very frustrating to use treatments that have no backing from science and which simply don't work. In desperation, after trying and failing to treat pimples with these misleading remedies, most will turn to expensive and often harmful powerful drugs.

Although tackling this misinformation is important on its own, it is not the primary reason why I started this book. As we'll see in the following few chapters, acne is a complicated disease with many causes, and it's highly unlikely that your first try at fixing your condition will be successful. I knew this when I first started treating my skin. I was aware that I had to go through many tests before I would find something that sticks. Although this trial-and-error tactic, alongside a complete lack of progress, was frustrating, it wasn't *the* most frustrating part of the whole experience. That part came after I started to take things into my own hands and research this disease to try and figure out why my skin hated me so much.

As I went my way through the medical research on this topic, I discovered things that were the complete opposite of what I knew about pimples. I was going down the wrong path and not treating what I should have. The most frustrating part of this whole experience wasn't that I was using recommended treatment options and not seeing results. Instead, I was misled about the causes of pimples, both by my own prejudices and the prejudices of those around me.

This book initially started as an experiment, a way for me to learn more about a disease that has riddled my entire adult life and which was beginning to take a serious toll on my mental health and self-confidence. But the more I read, the more confused I became, as the medical research on this topic told a different story from what I knew about pimples, and indeed about what most dermatologists recommend for treatment. At some point, I knew that I had to put these learnings into a book so others can learn from my mistakes.

Acne has existed with humans for almost as long as humans have existed. No one is safe from this disease, neither world leaders, emperors, pop stars, and, least of all, us ordinary people. Ancient Greek and Roman philosophers would obsess over the origin and treatment for this disease, laying the foundation of our understanding of acne. Although we've pondered about pimples for a long time, we're no closer to eradicating this disease than were our ancestors. No nation escapes zits (well, almost no nation, as we'll see later in this book). What's more, in recent years, it looks like the incidence rate of acne keeps growing, becoming a global problem that costs us billions to fix.

This disease seems universal and looks to be an inescapable part of puberty and growing up. At first glance, it might look like an easy problem to fix, as most of us have some basic understanding of how pimples form. Pores become clogged and get inflamed. To prevent it, you just need to stop these pore blockages from forming. As a result, most of us will turn to obsessively clean our faces, spending money we don't have on creams and lotions we don't need. Companies know this and know how desperate we can feel when we simply want to look decent. But very rarely do these expensive treatments truly work, and they don't help with the root cause either. An industry fueled by desperation can only flourish, which is why the dermatology business is worth billions of dollars today.

Treating acne is mostly a case of trial and error. This is how I started treating this disease, and I'm sure how many of you started as well. My first attempts at clearing my skin involved trying various creams and techniques to keep my face clean. I moved onto a strict washing routine, twice daily, once in the morning and once before bed. I changed my pillowcase religiously and never allowed anything dirty to touch my face, especially not my phone. I even developed a phobia of touching my face with my greasy fingers, which still persists even now that my acne is gone.

When this failed, I moved onto lotions with active ingredients and which were scientifically proven to work. Desperation fueled my irrationality, and I even bought creams that were banned where I live for having too many side effects. Alas, this failed as well. I was becoming hopeless, and my self-worth plummeted. As a last resort, I turned towards professional help, but regrettably, this was also was a trial and error process.

After a visit to the dermatologists and after spending a large lump of money that I didn't have, I came back home with a bag full of creams. These didn't work either. After researching the active ingredients of these "professional treatments," I became aware that these were nothing more than more expensive versions of stuff I was already using. I then connected the dots and figured out that the products I bought were the exact products advertised in the dermatologist's cabinet. Talk about conflict of interest.

At that point, I become so frustrated that I started to do research on my own. I couldn't believe that a disease so widespread and so debilitating wasn't cured yet. With an industry worth so much and with a disorder that seems simple to fix, it was hard for me to believe that we didn't find a way to prevent these pore blockages from happening. I expected to find the holy grail in some obscure medical journal that explains why we get pimples and how to cure them. Although this is partly true, as I delved deeper into the subject, it became apparent that acne's actual causes are much more complicated and, indeed, scary.

I got a good wake-up call as I read more about this topic. After a few late nights going through medical journals, it became apparent that acne is not just a disease of the face but one of the body. Mother Nature would never give us such a handicap when growing up, a time when we are at our most vulnerable and when social ties are crucial to healthy growth. Mother Nature would also never give us long-lasting scars in places that are crucial to socializing and bonding with others. That's because nature never gave us pimples. This disease is as human-made as any other modern disease, like the cancer brought by smoking or heart disease brought by over-indulgence.

Acne is not some inescapable part of our life that we have to get through the best that we can, and which we have to manage continuously using expensive creams. There are regions on Earth that have zero recorded cases of pimples at any age. This is not because they have some superhuman abilities or lead some expensive lifestyle. Quite the opposite. These superhumans that never get zits are what we consider "primitive tribes" that lack access to modern facilities, technology, and food. How do these people who don't use commercial lotions or acne drugs have such clear skin?

The answer to this is also the reason why acne is more than just a superficial disease. Acne doesn't stem from our inability to keep clean but from imbalances within us that affect the wellbeing of the entire body.

The scary part is that these imbalances don't affect only our skin. Acne is just the most visible part, but it's definitely not the most concerning. The same imbalances that give rise to acne are also linked with other, more serious diseases, including diabetes, various forms of cancers, neurodegenerative diseases, and many more. Because of this, it's paramount to treat the underlying imbalances instead of focusing on just our faces. If our treatment only goes skin deep, then the health improvements will also be superficial, paving the way for more severe health problems down the line. Because of this, I hope that by the end of this book, you will see that acne is actually a blessing and not a curse, as it's a mirror within our self, that helps us reflect on our overall wellbeing.

This contrast between the perceived and the actual causes of pimples can make acne a frustrating disease. It's frustrating because it seems an easy problem to fix and almost always thought to be caused by a lack of personal hygiene. It was frustrating to me to hear advice such as: "stop touching your face," "wash more often," or even "change your pillowcase at least twice a week." As we'll see later in this book, how often you wash your face or what comes into contact with your skin has very little to do with acne, if at all. The reason why we get acne is, unsatisfyingly, complicated, and it can't be distilled down to just one simple remedy. I'm sure there are anecdotes out there from people doing *this* simple trick that eliminated their acne forever. However, this disease is very rarely caused by just a single factor. Hence why there is no silver bullet (apart from medication, but even that involves some trial and error).

Don't get me wrong. I'm a pragmatist, and I'm all for quick fixes that can treat this debilitating disease and help us regain our lives. I have nothing against using pharmaceuticals to treat pimples, as I am well aware of just how damaging this disease is to our mental health. But, if you want to go one step further and understand why our skin hates us so, then I encourage you to read through the rest of the chapters with an open mind. As I mentioned previously, acne is a disease not of the face but of the body. We, humans, are complicated machinery. If one thing goes wrong in one part of the body, very rarely does that problem stay isolated. If one thing breaks, then many things break at the same time, and our skin is just one cog of a complex apparatus that must be kept in running order.

This book is structured into chapters that tackle specific myths about acne and why they might be true or false. Most of us have heard of these myths, and they mostly revolve around our diet or stressful activities. If you have acne, I'm sure you have "triggers" – like spicey food or chocolate – that you know for sure will give you pimples. We'll explore these myths throughout this book while also looking at the science that can explain why certain things can be bad for our skin and what really goes on inside us that makes us more likely to break out.

TABLE OF CONTENTS

INTRODUCTION

In Western countries, between 40% and 54% of adult men and women suffer from some form of acne. This number reaches as high as 95% in adolescence, making it the world's 8th largest affliction [1]. There were 645 million worldwide sufferers in 2010, more than the entire population of the US. And that number keeps growing every year.

It's not as fatal as cancer or heart disease, but it's definitely a debilitating illness. Studies have shown that people suffering from acne can have a reduced quality of life, including showing symptoms of depression, anxiety, anger, and low self-esteem [2] [3]. The fact that most people get acne during their teenage years, a time when we're more likely to be traumatized for life due to teasing and bullying, will amplify any negative experiences produced by this disease, causing it to become a burden for life. The physical scars might heal, but the mental ones will not.

Seeing as this disease is so common and impacts the mental health of so many people in the world, then surely, we have found a way to eradicate it completely by now?

The acne drug industry was estimated to be worth 15.45 billion US dollars in 2018 and is thought to grow to 20.48 billion US dollars by 2025 [4] (for comparison, that's almost as much as the GDP of Iceland). The fact that acne's prevalence is growing globally, especially in developing countries, means that this industry will continue to expand in the foreseeable future. Acne might be a burden on humanity, but it is certainly profitable for corporations. Cynics might argue that, with this much money involved, treating the underlying disease is not a priority to big corporations, as it might dry off their revenue stream. We have a pretty good understanding of what causes acne and how to prevent it, but programs that educate the general population are lacking. Think about how many times you have seen a commercial on TV on some new cream that will guarantee you'll have smooth skin, compared to infomercials on how to prevent this disease altogether. Although there is little evidence that hygiene plays a role in acne growth, this myth is still widespread among the general population [5]. The money is in treating pimples and not prevention.

Common acne treatments include topical ointments and creams like benzoyl peroxide or azelaic acid, which kill the acne-promoting bacteria that live on our skin; and oral medication that targets other pathways, like reducing oily skin or reducing the risk of inflammation when pores become blocked. In 2016 alone, Accutane – a popular drug administered for severe acne cases – was generating 1.2 billion US dollars in revenue yearly [6]. This drug has since been retracted, with the official claim that "it no longer makes business sense." However, it was also involved in several lawsuits regarding potential side-effects, including causing Crohn's disease and other inflammatory bowel disorders [7], indicating that there might be other reasons for its retraction.

Do these drugs work? In short, yes.

Today, the two most commonly prescribed treatments for acne are Benzoyl Peroxide, usually found as a topical gel in strengths of 2.5% to 10%; and Isotretinoin, which is ingested orally.

Benzoyl Peroxide works by killing the acne-promoting bacteria that live on our skin, usually on the face, and it is used to treat only mild to moderate acne forms. You might find this stuff either in cleansers or gels, usually mixed with some other ingredients like salicylic acid or sulfur, to increase the treatment's effectiveness. You will also find it in various concentrations, ranging from 2.5% to 10%, although there's no real evidence to support that higher strength gels work better than lower strength ones [8].

Benzoyl Peroxide is also one medication that can be bought over the counter, making it one of the most common and accessible acne treatments. Although, only some countries allow it to be purchased without a prescription (most notably in the United States). If you live in Europe, you can only get this treatment after visiting the doctor's office.

Several studies have shown that Benzoyl Peroxide is effective in treating mild to moderate forms of acne. One example is a randomized, controlled trial of 458 patients with varying acne severity levels, which were given gels with concentrations of 2.5% or 5% gels of this medication. The patients were followed for 52 weeks to assess if the number of active inflammations goes down after applying the cream. As early as the 2-week mark, both groups saw a decrease in lesion count by 30-35% compared to the baseline. At the end of the 54 weeks, both groups saw a reduction in pimples by 75-80% [9]. In short, it works.

Another popular drug on our list, isotretinoin (the active ingredient in Accutane), works in a slightly different way. If you're a long-time sufferer of acne, you have probably already performed some research into what causes acne and how you can treat it. You might already know that acne forms when sebum (the oily substance on our face) is combined with dead skill cells to create a mixture that clogs skin pores. Any bacteria trapped inside these chambers causes an inflammatory response from our skin, producing the dreaded pimples. Benzoyl Peroxide works by killing the bacteria which might get trapped in these cavities. In contrast, Isotretinoin works by stopping the sebum production altogether by targeting the glands that secrete it. If there's no sebum, then there's nothing to clog skin pores, thus preventing the formation of pimples altogether.

Similar to Benzoyl Peroxide, Isotretinoin has also shown positive results in clinical trials. In another randomized, placebo-controlled study, patients were split into two groups: one receiving 5mg of Isotretinoin daily for 16 weeks, with another group receiving a simple placebo. After as little as four weeks on this treatment, the group receiving Isotretinoin saw a decrease in lesion count compared to the placebo. After 16 weeks on Isotretinoin, patients had 69% fewer pimples when compared to the baseline [10]. And the best part about isotretinoin is that you don't have to take it continuously to eliminate acne completely. In contrast, Benzoyl Peroxide needs to be taken every day for as long as you are at risk of developing acne. Otherwise, the acne-promoting bacteria will regrow, and pimples will start forming once more. However, a 2-month treatment with Isotretinoin is usually enough to have clear skin forever.

There is a pretty well-established procedure for treating acne. First, dermatologists will recommend a series of drugs to try until one is found that works, depending on the severity of acne and the effectiveness of other tested drugs. This means that dermatologists will prescribe a standard treatment program, minimizing the risk of being overly aggressive from the start, thus reducing potential side effects. Although many drugs can stop acne, the list of active ingredients that power these medications is relatively small. For this reason, you'll get more bang for your buck if you use generics instead of name brands, as long as you make sure the active ingredient is still the same.

Benzoyl peroxide and isotretinoin are only two out of many medications that have shown promising results in reducing acne symptoms. Both medicines were scientifically proven to stop acne, so why not simply go with this route from the get-go?

The answer to this is twofold, and part one is based on intuition. The human body has evolved over hundreds of thousands of years to optimize our quality of life and maximize our reproduction chances based on our environment. Why then have we evolved into a state in which we are practically disfigured in critical moments of our life? Indeed, there are still abnormal health conditions caused by inherited or mutated genes passed down from our ancestors, but these conditions remain rare for the general population.

On the other hand, acne has an almost 100% incidence rate in certain nations, and it's implausible to think that Mother Nature hasn't developed a way to prevent pimples after so many generations of humans. It's much more likely that acne is a human-made disease, similar to the lung cancer caused by smoking, making it a new development rather than an illness that has always existed in humans. There are regions on Earth where acne is almost non-existent, as we'll see later in this book. If acne is truly a manifestation of something more serious gone haywire in our body, are we treating only the superficial symptoms instead of the underlying problem?

The second reason why pharmaceutical drugs are likely not the best treatment option for acne is tied to the following list of side effects. Can you guess which medicine has them?

Skin dryness, itching, burning sensation, peeling, flaking, irritation, and redness.

If you've guessed "Benzoyl Peroxide," you'd be right.

What about the following list?

Back pain, joint pain, muscle pain, dry nose, dry skin, dry lips, dry mouth, dry eyes, nosebleeds, cracks in the corner of mouths, peeling or cracking skin, inflammation of the whites of the eyes, drowsiness, dizziness, nervousness, changes in fingernails or toenails, swelling of eyelids, swelling of lips, upset stomach, thinning of hair, depression, low energy.

You've likely found the pattern, but the previous list presents possible side effects of the isotretinoin drug.

In the above list, we forgot to mention one other potential side effect: death! Several studies link Isotretinoin with an increase in risk for pancreatitis, a potentially fatal disease. These studies found several patients that started developing pancreatitis some weeks after beginning acne treatment with isotretinoin [11]. It's a rare side effect, and the exact causes leading to this disease are currently unknown. Still, patients who are prescribed isotretinoin are now also recommended to undertake regular tests to measure levels of triglycerides (an early indicator of pancreatitis), which can potentially catch serious adverse effects early on.

You might argue that any drug will have its side effects. Before prescribing a treatment, a medical practitioner will usually balance the positive impact with the potential side effects the medicine might have. This is why the standard procedure for treating acne involves first prescribing almost benign medication (like ordinary face cleansers), then moving to ingredients that are more active but with potentially few side effects (like benzoyl peroxide or azelaic acid), and then finally moving to the riskiest but the likeliest to succeed drugs (isotretinoin). The catch with this scheme is that the more severe acne you have, the more emotional strain you will be under, making you more likely to accept treatments with worse side effects. Unfortunately, these patients will have the highest burden on their life, both from acne itself and the remedy against this disease.

If only there were another way…

There is another way

Remember the statistic we presented in the introduction that mentioned that 79% to 95% of the adolescent population suffers from some form of acne? In reality, this high incidence of acne exists only in *some* nations. There are areas of the globe in which acne is virtually non-existent at any age.

The highest acne rates are observed in countries that we commonly referred to as *Western nations*. If you look at the entire globe, acne is becoming more common as a whole [12]. However, it is believed that the reason why acne rates are increasing each year is that the Western way of life is reaching more and more countries, which are beginning to adopt dietary and lifestyle changes specific to Western nations. This is quite a bold statement, considering that, traditionally, acne is associated with hygiene and not diet or lifestyle. One would expect that Western nations have a lower incidence of acne due to their obsession with cleanliness. But, the reality is quite the opposite – primarily countries with higher socio-economical status have a higher incidence of acne, and not the other way around.

One way for you to check these claims yourself and verify acne incidence rates specific to your region is to use the *Global Burden of Disease* database. This database is run by the World Health Organization and provides free information about a broad range of mortality and disability causes from all regions of Earth. We can use this database to break down acne rates by country, year, economic status, or other factors. You can easily visualize this database through the following website: https://vizhub.healthdata.org/gbd-compare/

If you plot the prevalence of acne broken down by year, you'll see that these illness rates are increasing only for some countries – most notably those that have recently had explosive economic growth. These include nations or regions such as India, South America, and some countries in Eastern Europe. Areas that we consider "developed nations," such as North America or Western Europe, have higher than average acne rates than the rest of the world. They have seen a slower increase in incidence in recent years, indicating that they have reached peak acne commonality. If you want to explore this data, you can start from the following link: http://ihmeuw.org/5047

These indicators are not proof that the Western way of life causes acne, but they do provide a valuable hint to start our research. When we think of Western civilizations, we usually envision certain lifestyle elements that might be linked with acne. These nations are associated with an above-average economic status and general well being, are more stressed by an overload of information and activities, eat less healthy foods (such as fast food, pre-packaged or heavily processed food), are generally more obese than average, and experience high levels of pollution. Any one of these markers can be a potential candidate for triggering acne, and each one has its own associated myth. Some people believe that chocolate will trigger pimples, others swear they break out after eating spicy food, while others are convinced that stressful life events are the caused for their acne. We will look at all of these common myths throughout this book.

How can we tell that something in the Western culture causes acne? Simple. We can compare acne rates between Western nations and those that are so unlike modern civilizations that they have virtually nothing in common. Thankfully, we have such examples. Some have been the center of numerous scientific studies due to their remoteness and simple way of life.

One such population is the inhabitants of the Kitavan island. This small region at the east of Papua New Guinea measures only 23 square kilometers, less than half of the Manhattan island. This island is part of a more extensive archipelago, called the Trobriand Islands, which, since the 70s, has shifted towards an economy based primarily on tourism and export. So it would be a stretch to say that modern life hasn't reached the inhabitants, especially considering we can find 360 pictures of the region on Google Maps. However, these islanders still live mostly traditional lives, on a diet consisting of fruits and vegetables sourced locally.

This aspect alone would be an interesting research point in understanding the way of life of early Homo sapiens, but what's truly remarkable about these inhabitants is their extraordinary health. Despite a fair share of older inhabitants, none show signs of dementia or poor memory. Medical experts with knowledge of the Kitavan island report no premature deaths due to cardiovascular disease, and EKG tests performed directly on the inhabitants confirmed the excellent overall heart health [13]. Kitavans also have low rates of obesity; on average, men had a BMI of 20, and women a BMI of 18 [14]. In comparison, in 2016, the average male American had a BMI of 29, and the average female 30 [15].

Because of their extraordinary health, Kitavans have been the subject of numerous studies linking their way of life to improved health. One reason why we believe Kitavans live healthier lives is due to their diet. They are traditional farmers, eating mostly plant-based foods (yam, sweet potato, taro, fruits, coconuts) and non-domesticated animals (like fish). Under 1% of their diet consists of what we consider "Western foods." They consume no dairy, alcohol, coffee, or tea.

Similarly, their intake of oils, margarine, cereals, and refined sugars is considerably lower than in Western nations. Because they live on a mostly plant-based diet, they eat more fiber, minerals, and vitamins compared to the average Western country [16]. Overall, the Kitavan diet differs by more than 30 nutrients from Western diets, mainly from their low consumption of salt and fatty foods, from the high ratio of omega-3 to omega-6 fatty acids, and from a low preponderance for sugary foods. Because of this, Kitavans are the perfect candidates for studies on the link between diet and various health conditions, including acne.

In 1990, a group of Swedish researchers visited the island in the hopes of findings connections between the dietary preferences of Kitavans and their health. Participating in the research team was Staffan Lindeberg, an associate professor now known for his extensive research on evolutionary health principles and the Kitava study. His work on the health benefits of following an early Homo sapiens diet was foundational. He also led multiple research projects, both on the field and through clinical trials on ancestral diet and lifestyle. The initial work done in the 90s gave him the early insights that projected his research throughout the rest of his career.

Lindeberg found that, out of the 1200 Kitavan subjects examined for dermatological conditions, none had acne. This included some 300 inhabitants aged 15 to 25 who are at high risk of developing this disease. If you were to perform the same survey in a typical Western nation, out of the 300 subjects, you would expect to find at least 120 which have active acne [1]. The fact that none of the inhabitants had pimples is truly remarkable, especially considering that they lacked modern acne treatments, such as Benzoyl Peroxide or isotretinoin.

These results were mirrored by other studies performed in similar regions of the globe, where Western culture is still absent. More notably is the research done on the Aché hunter-gatherer tribes in eastern Paraguay, which, unlike Kitavans, lead a much more active lifestyle. This tribe initially inhabited a region of 20,000 km^2 in an area between the Paraguay and Paraná rivers, in which they gathered their food through hunting and foraging. However, since the first contact with Western nations in the 1970s, their active region was reduced to just a few dedicated reserves of less than 50 km^2. Despite this, their diet is still very similar to that of early Homo sapiens, with an abundance of wild, foraged foods. Only 8% of their diet consists of procured Western foods; the vast majority of energy intake comes from cultivated plants (sweet manioc, peanuts, maize, rice) and wild game.

Similar to the Kitavan study, no cases of active acne were recorded in the Aché population throughout a two-year examination period involving 115 patients. Of these inhabitants, only a single male had acne scars but no active pimples. This study also included inhabitants at high risk of developing acne – girls and boys younger than 25 years old – but no acne cases were recorded in this segment either [1].

Can we conclude that diet is the sole reason why Kitavans and Aché hunter-gatherers have such low acne rates?

Although some of these tribes are significantly more physically active than the typical Westerner, previous research has found no strong link between physical exercise and acne [17]. Genetics might play a role; familial studies indicate that acne is partly hereditary. If a first-degree relative has acne (like your parents or siblings), you're much more likely to develop this disease as well [18]. However, genetic aspects are unlikely to play a large role in the results found on Kitava and Aché inhabitants, since other native South American and Pacific descends have high acne incidence rates if they switch to a Western lifestyle [1].

Regressing to the lifestyle of early Homo sapiens is not an option anymore – we would sacrifice too much to rid ourselves of acne. However, maybe we don't need to change everything about our lives to improve our health.

The rest of this book explores the science behind what we know works against acne and what doesn't, how true are the common myths surrounding acne, and which of the dietary and environmental factors particular to Kitavans give them their extraordinary health. In 1985, Stanley Boyd Eaton and Melvin Konner published a controversial article in the New England Journal of Medicine, which stated that we are genetically programmed to consume pre-agricultural foods because we are biologically similar to our primitive ancestors. By swaying far from the "optimal diet," our modern way of life has given rise to the biggest killers in Western nations, including heart disease, diabetes, obesity, and cancer. In the rest of the book, we will find out if these principles apply to acne as well.

We will initially explore how acne is formed and what are the mechanical aspects of pimples. We will understand what pores are, what causes them to become clogged, and why they turn into inflamed pimples. Afterward, we will summarize the research done on acne risk factors to see how we can prevent this disease. We will look at specific food items, lifestyle, and environmental aspects that are thought to influence acne. Finally, in the later chapters, we will consolidate our learnings into one big picture to have a broad understanding of how acne works and how to prevent it.

But, before we delve deeper into the subject, it should be prefaced that acne is a complicated disease that has many causes. There is no silver bullet that magically makes pimples disappear overnight. Although we have a pretty good understanding of what leads to acne, the solutions involve long-term lifestyle changes that can take months to take effect.

Considering that acne has such a strong influence over our mental and general wellbeing, it's perfectly understandable if you need a quick fix using modern medicine. However, it doesn't have to be an either-or situation. You can still use pharmaceutical treatments to rid yourself of acne quickly and regain control of your life but still apply some of the long-term changes described in this book to fix the underlying disease instead of just the manifestation.

Some of the factors that we know trigger acne are also associated with other, more severe conditions. These include various forms of cancer, diabetes, and neurodegeneration [19]. Most illnesses don't affect just a single organ — failure is systematic throughout our body. The cause of acne is simply an imbalance, one which has long-reaching ramifications. You can think of pimples as an early warning signal that something has gone astray in ourselves. It's our responsibility to listen to these warnings and not just hide them.

CHAPTER SUMMARY

- Acne is an increasingly common disease, affecting 79% to 95% of adolescents.

- Acne rates are rising globally. The highest prevalence of acne is seen in Western regions, like North America or Western Europe. This observation has given rise to theories that acne is a human-made disease caused by factors specific to Western civilization (diet, pollution, stress, etc.).

- Hunter-gatherer societies have no recorded cases of acne.

- Modern treatments are highly effective in treating acne; however, they usually come with severe side effects, creating the need for alternative therapies that are safer and cheaper.

- It's believed that acne is just a manifestation of more severe imbalances in our bodies. By treating acne instead of the underlying problem, we risk developing more dangerous illnesses in the future.

WHAT IS ACNE?

Acne has existed with humans for at least as long as recorded history. It's unknown who was the first to succumb to this disease, but the earliest mention of acne dates back to Egyptian times. In the Eberus Papyrus – a series of ancient Egyptian papers describing medicinal practices – the term "aku-t" was used to describe a skin condition that manifested as inflamed swellings and was later translated as "boils, blains, and sores" [20].

Egyptian medicine is one of the oldest that we know but also one of the most primitive. Although ancient Egyptians were aware of the importance nutrition plays in human health, they also based their treatments on superstition and magic. Amulets were a popular treatment option for certain diseases, as were incantations and magical spells. Many of the healers were also part priests of the Sekhmet god – the Egyptian goddess of healing.

Although most ancient Egyptian treatments were based more on superstition than scientific rigor, some plant-based medicine options survived even to this date. Sulfur was first used during the time of Cleopatra (69-30 BC) and is still commercialized as an added ingredient in face creams in modern acne treatments. Honey was also a popular treatment for acne in ancient Egyptian times, being one of the most used herbal remedies at that time [21].

Because Egyptians kept rigorous writing documents of standard medical practices, we can deduce that even Pharaohs succumbed to this disease by analyzing the items with which they were buried and comparing them with typical acne treatments from that time. For example, we can guess that Tutankhamun likely had acne until the day he died. His tomb contained items commonly used as acne remedies at that time, documented in the Eberus Papyrus [20].

The earliest known mention of the word "acne" dates back to the ancient Greek writing of Aetius Amidinos, a Byzantine physician. His work derived the term "acne" from the Greek word "acme," meaning "point" or "spot" [20]. At that time, however, treatment options for acne were still primitive. Physicians recommended honey to soften acne lesions and soap for the more stubborn spots [22]. Before the term "acne" was coined, ancient Greeks used a different word to describe this disease, derived from the name "tovoot" – meaning "the first growth of beard" [22]. Because of this, Greeks from that era likely knew that acne is more common during puberty, a notion that holds to this day.

It wasn't until the invention of the microscope, some one thousand years after the time of Amidinos, that we started to really understand what causes pimples.

Marcello Malpighi, an Italian biologist who lived in the 17th century, is considered the founder of microscopic anatomy. He made several discoveries only possible through the use of a microscope: he was the first to detect capillaries in animals, the first to see red blood cells, and also discovered that invertebrates use trachea for breathing instead of lungs. He was also the first to see the tiny glands at the base of skin pores that secrete sebum.

Some years later, a French professor of Medicine named Jean Astruc used the term *sebaceous glands* to describe these glands, a phrase which stuck to this day [20]. The name *sebaceous* is derived from the Latin word "sebaceus," meaning tallow or grease. Astruc chose this word likely because these glands produce an oily substance similar in texture to melted animal fats. We now call this secreted mixture *sebum*.

At the beginning of the 19th century, the basis of our understanding of acne was set. We now could see that the skin is riddled with tiny chambers through which hairs stick out. Most of these hairs are invisible until you look closely, but they are present throughout our body: on our face, buttocks, back, and arms. Women have these tiny hairs as well, despite what they might try to convince you otherwise.

At the base of the small chambers, glands exist which secrete the sebum substance. Usually, sebum travels up the hair shaft to reach our skin's outer layer, helping to lubricate and provide an initial barrier against bacteria and other foreign pathogens. However, this same process that lubricates our skin can cause pimples if the pores that secrete sebum become clogged.

Sebum secretion doesn't stop if there's nowhere for it to go. If pores are blocked, glands will continue to build pressure by continuously pumping sebum. In certain people, this build-up of tension doesn't lead to anything too severe. For these lucky people, the outer layer of the clog will oxidize when in contact with air, turning dark in color. These non-inflamed blocked pores are called blackheads as they turn black when oxidized by the oxygen in the atmosphere. They are easily treatable with an ordinary face scrub. However, in some people, the pressure inside skin pores can become so great that the outer skin layer ruptures, spewing the accumulated sebum deeper within our skin. As bad as this sounds, this is still not enough to produce the inflamed blemishes we associate with acne. There's one more missing ingredient.

In the 20th century, dermatologists had some initial hints that some unknown catalyst plays a significant role in acne development. When looking at the skin of some human patients, they found unusually large quantities of some chemicals that we can't produce naturally. The presence of these substances could only be explained by some undiscovered enzyme that can break down sebum into these chemicals. We now know that this catalyst is a special kind of bacteria that lives on our skin and which eats sebum, breaking it down into the raw substances initially discovered in the 20th century [23].

When the skin ruptures inside a blocked pore, not only does sebum gets pushed deeper into our skin, but it also injects certain species of bacteria that thrive on sebum. One, in particular, called *Cutibacterium acnes* (C. acnes), feeds primarily on sebum and is found in abundance throughout our skin.

As we'll see later in this book, C. acnes is usually beneficial to us – it helps build an acidic layer that sits on top of our skin. This protective layer can kill off harmful pathogens, being the first line of defense against many diseases. However, when bacteria get trapped inside blocked skin pores, they are free to multiply, preferring conditions devoid of oxygen. Once the skin ruptures and bacteria are released in our skin, the immune system activates to trigger inflammation, creating the dreaded pimples.

This is an over-simplified view of how acne is formed, but we will improve our understanding throughout this book. For now, it is sufficient to know that pimples are created when sebum and bacteria are released deep within our skin, causing the immune and inflammatory systems to activate.

As you read through the previous paragraph, an idea likely popped into your head: what if, to prevent pimples, we dissolve the cap which forms at the top of our skin pores? Indeed, this is how some acne treatments work, including some of the earliest known remedies for this disease.

Ancient Romans loved their baths infused with sulfur, as they believed this mineral possesses healing properties. Sulfur reacts with the amino acids present on our skin's outer layer to form hydrogen sulfide – a highly corrosive substance known for its smell, similar to rotten eggs. This compound interacts with the binding agents that hold pore clogs together. In a way, sulfur acts as a drain cleaner for our skin, removing pore blockages before they become inflamed pimples [22]. Other modern treatments work in a similar way, including salicylic acid [24].

Although some of these treatments have been proven to be somewhat effective [25], they are not very efficient. As you can imagine, to prevent pimples from forming, you would have to continuously apply sulfur-based lotions for as long as you are at risk. Once you stop using treatments that dissolve pore blockages, these clogs will start reappearing and, with them, acne as well. To be more efficient in treating acne, we would have to prevent these obstructions altogether. As the saying goes, prevention is better than cure.

To understand why pores become blocked in the first place, we will first make our way through an analogy. Imagine a syringe initially filled with nothing but air. The plunger from such a syringe will move quite freely when you press it. However, if you then fill the syringe with water and try pressing the plunger again, you will feel some resistance. Even so, it's still quite manageable, and you can easily squeeze the water out.

But what happens when you fill the syringe with honey? Pressing the plunger will become much harder, as honey doesn't flow as freely compared with water or wair. If you swap honey with an even thicker substance, like tar, it becomes near impossible to push the plunger anymore. All three materials — water, honey, tar — are classified as liquids, but they have different physical properties, making some flow easier while others harder. The property of a liquid to resist movement is called *viscosity* and is the primary catalyst that causes blockages to occur in our pores.

The same principles of liquid thickness apply to sebum as well. If sebum flows freely (has low viscosity), then it will easily pass through skin pores. However, if sebum has high viscosity — similar to tar in a syringe — it will resist movement, stopping the flow altogether. If sebum is sufficiently thick, then blockages will occur, building pressure inside pores, ultimately leading to inflammation.

Sebum is not a uniform substance — it is comprised of many different compounds. At a high level, substances from 7 classes of chemicals form sebum: Glycerides, Free Fatty Acids, Wax Esters, Squalene, Cholesterol Esters, and Cholesterol [26]. In total, sebum is made of tens of different chemicals, each one with different physical properties. Certain mixtures of these chemicals flow easier, keeping our skin in optimal health, while others have high viscosity, causing pore blockages. More so, certain compounds can even promote bacterial growth or encourage unnecessary inflammation. Keeping the right balance between these substances is key to acne prevention.

How do we keep the optimal composition of sebum? That is a complicated topic, one which will be the basis of this book. Many factors control how much sebum is produced and the final mixture composition. Not all of these factors are known or well understood, but we have made good progress in recent years in unraveling the complex system governing acne.

As it turns out, sebum isn't the only bad guy. Acne is a disease with a multitude of causes. Sebum production – although a crucial player – isn't the only factor. Inflammation, bacterial growth, and excessive dead skin cells also conspire to give us pimples. Some acne variants are even created when our skin is exposed to highly reactive substances resulting from air pollution, without pores ever becoming blocked.

Thankfully, as our understanding of acne grows, we now know that all of these risk factors are controlled by only a handful of key players. As we'll see later in the book, acne is not a genetic condition but one which is caused by an imbalance in these core players. To understand who they are and how to control them, we will go through common myths surrounding acne to understand what is the actual science behind these risk factors and why certain foods or lifestyle choices can harm our skin. You will notice a pattern emerging in which certain metabolic processes will appear in almost all acne pathways. And where better to start our journey than with one of the most addictive substances on earth: sugar [27].

CHAPTER SUMMARY

- Acne forms when obstructions to skin pores cause ruptures to our skin, spilling a mixture of sebum, dead skin cells, and bacteria in our skin. Once our body detects these intruders, it will trigger local inflammation, producing pimples.

- Some acne treatments dissolve skin pore clogs (such as sulfur), but they have to be used continuously for as long as you are at risk.

- Although acne is a complicated disease, only a few key players control the multitude of factors that can lead to pimples. We will explore them throughout the rest of the book.

Part I

DIET

HIGH GLYCEMIC FOODS

No one can deny the addictive nature of sugar. It is so habit-forming that it is used ubiquitously in almost everything we eat, from soft drinks to canned baked beans. Despite its popularity, there is growing evidence that overeating sugar can be harmful to our health, leading to obesity, cardiovascular diseases, type 2 diabetes, and non-alcoholic fatty liver disease [28]. Sugar has become such an epidemic that the World Health Organization now recommends reducing the quantity of consumed sugar to be less than 5% of daily caloric intake [29].

Despite these warnings, the average Westerner still consumes three times the recommended daily dose [30]. Although it's not the biggest food-related killer of Westerners (that spot can be attributed to animal products and processed junk [31] [32] [33]), sugar deserves special attention. And, seeing as it impacts so many organs and bodily functions, it's entirely reasonable to expect that it might also have some influence over our skin.

Sugar is part of a larger food group called *carbohydrates*, commonly known for being the primary energy source of the human body. Because carbs are so energy-dense, they are also famous for making us fat, as they can cause us to reach our daily calorie limit quite quickly. Indeed, carbs are primarily broken down by the human body into fuel for our cells. However, they also serve other important functions, including being used as building blocks for molecular structures (such as for RNA).

Carbohydrates are essential to us as they are one of the larger nutrients groups the human body needs to function correctly, alongside proteins, fats, and fiber. This means that it's not exactly wise to stop eating carbs altogether. There is evidence which suggests that following a low-carb diet for prolonged times can lead to cardiovascular complication and bone health deterioration [34]. People eating a low-carb diet also consume fewer vegetables and fruits (as these are also rich in sugars), meaning they consume fewer essential nutrients that protect us against a multitude of diseases. As a result, people on a low-carb diet are also at higher risk of developing various cancers [34].

Although carbs are mainly beneficial, not all food items in this group are equally valuable. There is increasing evidence that links carbs with acne, whereby people who eat lots of sugary foods will tend to develop more acne.

In China, one group of scientists asked over 8000 students to describe their typical weekly diet. The participants were asked to fill out a questionnaire about their soft drinks intake – such as carbonated sugary drinks, sweetened tea, and other flavored drinks. This data was then matched up with acne prevalence among the participants. The researchers found that drinking *any* amount of sugary beverage was associated with a higher risk of developing acne. The effect was most potent when sugary drinks were consumed more than seven times a week.

Interestingly, the occasional intake of fruit-flavored drinks (1-2 times per week) had a mild positive effect, reducing acne in some patients. This observation may be due to the protective nature of fruits in general, but the association was pretty weak either way. Very high consumption of sugar through soft drinks showed a significant association with acne, particularly if the quantity of consumed sugar exceeded 100g per day [38].

Similar results were found in another epidemiological study, this time performed on identical and fraternal twins. What better way to validate if diet or the environment has any effect on our skin than to do so on people who have identical or similar sets of genes?

Every year, on the first full weekend in August, a series of festivities are held in Twinsburg, Ohio, to celebrate biological twins. Although it is primarily a time of celebration, it's also an excellent opportunity for scientists to get insights from the largest gathering of twins on Earth. This festival regularly receives 2,000 participants each year, and, in 2016, a group of researchers used this opportunity to question the participants on their dietary habits.

The researchers found that, in a single pair of siblings, the twin which consumed more sugar also had more pimples [39]. Seeing as the genetic information between the twins was identical or extremely similar, these results indicate that acne is not an entirely hereditary disease and that diet and the environment do play an important role.

The association between sugar and acne is generally well established, being confirmed by many other epidemiological studies [40] [41] [42]. It's now well known that people who eat more fast carbs or sugary foods also tend to develop more pimples. Yet, although the link between the two is strong, it does not necessarily mean that eating sugary foods will cause acne. The two are indeed connected, but we don't know for sure if one causes the other. It can be just as likely that people who can afford sugary foods can also afford other foods known to cause acne. This faulty reasoning is commonly known as the *correlation trap*.

My favorite example of a correlation trap starts with a simple observation about wind speeds. If you gaze out the window on a random day, you might see and hear the wind gushing more than average. On other days, the wind is perfectly still, without so much as a light breeze. You also notice that the movement of the trees is closely linked with how windy it is. On particularly stormy days, the trees sway more as the wind blows. While on calm days with no air currents, the trees are also perfectly still. You then naturally conclude that trees cause the wind to move faster.

Obviously, this is incorrect. We know from past experiences that the wind is the one that makes the trees sway, not the other way around. But, judging only from our observation that higher wind speeds are correlated with the foliage movement, there would be no way for us to know the causation direction. We would need to test both claims: remove all the trees from a nearby field to see if the wind continues to blow stronger on some days, and also remove the wind (or perform the observation in a region without too many air currents) to see if the trees continue to sway.

To definitively say whether sugar causes acne, we would need to take one group of acne patients and change their diet for some weeks to see if, by reducing sugar intake, their acne improves. This is exactly what one group of Australian researchers set out to do. They recruited male students aged 15 to 25 and split them into two groups. The first group was asked to follow a low-carb diet for the duration of the experiment, while the other group was instructed to follow a high-carb diet. More specifically, the low-sugar diet consisted of around 25% protein, 45% low glycemic-index carbohydrates, and 30% fats.

After seeing the previous list of nutrients assigned to the low-carb diet, you might be wondering why carbohydrates were in such a high proportion, considering that the purpose of the experiment was to decrease blood sugar levels. The answer to this anomaly is that not all carbs are created equal.

Carbs differ in their ability to give either a large or a small dose of molecular energy. Because of this, some carbs are good for our health, making us feel full for longer without too much energy intake. In contrast, other carbs are potentially dangerous, delivering a sudden rush of energy, but which doesn't last long, leading to more cravings and more sugar intake.

Glucose is the primary molecule that transports energy throughout our body, and most carbs are converted into glucose as soon as they are ingested. This way, the energy stored in these foods can be digested and transported in the bloodstream, giving fuel to our cells. Because it doesn't have to go through any significant chemical transformations before being usable, glucose is the preferred energy source of most living things. However, our body can use other nutrients for energy, like proteins and fat. Otherwise, we would starve quite quickly, as glucose reserves in humans are relatively low compared to fat or protein sources. The average human stores about 500g of glucose [35], compared to 27Kg of muscle mass, and 18Kg of fat [36]. The human body can breakdown these other macro-nutrients for energy, but ultimately everything is still converted into glucose before being used by cells.

The amount of glucose a particular food item releases is measured through its *glycemic index* and *glycemic load.* Foods with a high glycemic <u>index</u> cause your blood glucose levels to spike to high values, as they release their energy very quickly. This number indicates what will be the maximum blood concentration level of glucose. Similarly, glycemic <u>load</u> measures what will be the total amount of glucose released after eating a particular food item.

In general, foods with a high glycemic index (like candy bars or sodas) will give you that sugar-rush immediately after consuming them, but they will also give you a sugar crash, as glucose levels eventually drop below the value you had before eating these foods. Similarly, foods with a low glycemic index make you feel full for longer, as the drop in glucose levels is more gradual.

Foods with a low GI [37] (GI under 50)	Foods with a high GI [37] (GI over 70)
• Barley (28)	• White wheat bread (75)
• Brown rice (50)	• Cornflakes (81)
• Apple (36)	• Potato (78)
• Orange (43)	• Ice cream (51)
• Vegetable soup (48)	• Rice milk (86)
• Chickpeas (28)	• Sodas (59)
• Kidney beans (24)	• Popcorn (65
• Soya beans (16)	
• Lentils (32)	

Although glucose is the primary energy transport molecule, it can't be used directly by our cells. First, it has to pass the outer cell membrane and then be converted into raw molecules that can act as fuel. Glucose is primarily used to move energy in the body but still has to go through several transformations before being used as energy.

Glucose also can't penetrate the cell membrane on its own; it needs some help in the form of a hormone called *insulin*, which makes the cell membrane permeable and lets glucose through. You've likely heard of this hormone from people who have diabetes. In healthy individuals, when blood glucose levels rise, the pancreas produces sufficient insulin to match the quantity of glucose, helping our cells get enough energy. However, in people with diabetes, the body either doesn't make enough insulin, or cells develop resistance to this hormone. If this happens, cell membranes won't be as permeable to glucose, meaning the host cell won't get enough energy to function correctly, leading to cell starvation and death.

For optimal health, the two molecules – glucose and insulin – have to be kept in constant balance. If there's too little insulin, then glucose can't be used as energy by the human body. Too much insulin will also be detrimental, as it triggers the over-usage of glucose, depleting energy reserves, leading to what is commonly known as low blood sugar.

The balance between the two molecules is also through to influence our skin, and this is precisely what the Australian group of researchers set out to verify. Although there are many different types of carbs, some will give a short burst of insulin, while others will release their energy more slowly.

In the Australian experiment, the low-sugar group was eating carbs, but they were of the variety that slowly releases their energy. For example, barley – which is still a carbohydrate – has a much lower glycemic index than white rice and even lower than refined white bread. As long as you choose foods with a low glycemic index, you can still consume a diet rich in carbohydrates without being subjected to the harmful effects of high glucose levels. You can find many resources online that will give the glycemic index and load for multiple food groups, but a starting point is at http://bit.ly/2TK9O4y

Both groups of participants consumed similar levels of calories each day. Even so, the low-sugar group reduced the average glycemic index of their foods from 59 to 47 by consuming only carbs with a glycemic index lower than 55.

The study itself took 12 weeks to complete. In the end, the researchers noticed that the group which ate only low-glycemic foods saw a decrease in inflamed and total pimple count compared to the baseline [43] (see Figure 1 - Low GI diet effect on acne). The results were pretty dramatic, as the group with an altered diet saw an almost 50% reduction in pimple count when compared with the baseline. The trendline also indicates that if the study had taken longer than the allocated 12 weeks, more significant improvements would have been seen. What's more, the same treatment group also lost 2.9 Kg in body weight on average, while control patients gained 0.5Kg, even if both groups consumed the same number of calories each day.

The researchers also found that both total glycemic index and load were inversely correlated with acne severely. The fewer carbs that were consumed by the patients, the greater the reduction in pimple count was. Interestingly, the study also found a link between saturated fats usage and acne. Similar to carbs, the patients who consumed fewer saturated fats had fewer pimples on average. We will come back to this topic later in the book.

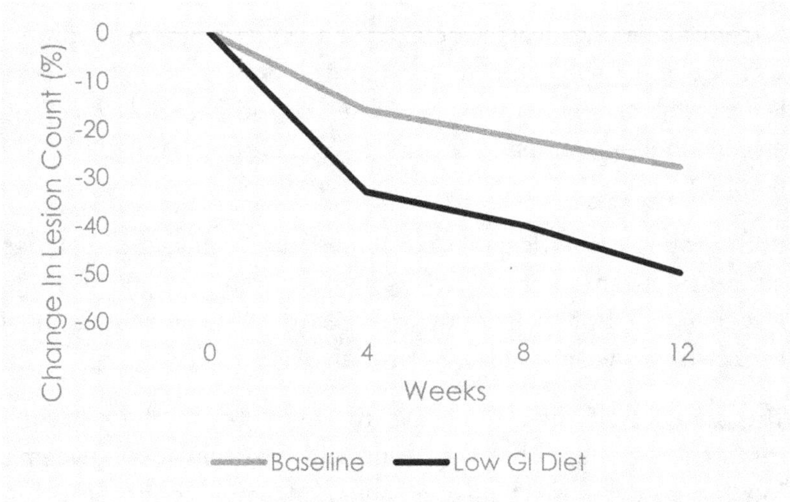

Figure 1 - Low GI diet effect on acne

What's strange about this experiment is that both the low-carb and baseline groups saw an improvement in acne. The explanation for this is likely that both groups of patients were prescribed a standard face washing routine at the beginning of the experiment. To account for different face-washing practices that the patients might have had before the trial, the researchers asked all participants to switch to a single consistent routine. This change in washing habits could have explained the improvement in the baseline group, as previous research indicates that simply washing your face twice a day can reduce acne symptoms [44]. The participants that did not clean their face regularly might have seen an improvement just by switching to this new routine.

Despite this anomaly, the study did show a relative improvement between the two groups, where individuals consuming foods with a lower glycemic index saw a reduction in their blood insulin levels and acne severity.

Other similar experiments confirmed these results. Another randomized control experiment measured the effectiveness of a low glycemic-index diet in reducing acne lesions, but this time for a 10-week trial. At the end of the study, the group eating fewer sugary food items saw a decrease in acne severity. The researchers also found that the size of the sebum-producing glands decreased and that fewer pro-inflammatory proteins were present in the skins of the patients following a low glycemic-index diet [45].

In another study, 31 patients were given either a low glycemic diet (only ate foods that had a glycemic-index lower than 55) or a standard diet for two weeks. Although the study was too short to prove that such a diet improves acne itself, the researchers did find a reduction in certain hormones known to cause acne [46].

The evidence supporting the idea that high sugar intake aggravates acne is quite overwhelming. Both epidemiological studies and more controlled experiments agree that eating sugary foods exacerbates acne. The more sugary foods you eat, the worse the acne gets. But, what could explain this effect?

Because sebum is a very fatty substance, one would expect that carbs (which have almost no fat) do not affect our skin. More so, to keep the same calorie intake, if one were to give up carbs completely, they would have to replace this food group with something else – probably fats or proteins. It would be natural to assume that this added dietary fat would make acne worse, considering that we would give more raw material for sebum to form. Yet, the evidence suggests quite the opposite.

The answer to this paradox lies in how sebum and sebum composition is regulated. Because sebum has high quantities of fatty molecules, it is controlled by the same factors that manage fat production in general.

The human body needs a way to regulate how much fat to burn for energy, when to make new fat reserves, and where to allocate fat. Because of this, humans have a master regulator of lipid production, which senses the nutritional state of our body, and makes decisions regarding how much and when to create new lipids. This regulator also controls sebum production, making it essential in our understanding of acne.

The master regulator of sebum

Our DNA is the central manual on how to build and maintain the human body. It encodes information on everything from how many limbs we have, the composition of our nails, and how predisposed we are to certain diseases. Some compare our DNA to a computer program; it provides instructions on how to execute commands relating to growth, survival, and prosperity. Because of this, the DNA also stores data about how likely we are to develop acne and how to create and maintain all the systems that might lead to acne. However, the analogy that the DNA is similar to a computer program falls apart at some point, as there is no central processor that reads commands from our DNA and executes them. The principle of how our DNA converts information into useful products is much simpler than this.

Proteins are one of the fundamental molecule groups that sustain life. They are used in everything from providing cell structure, information transportation, fighting off infections, and even creating other proteins. Although complex in structure, these molecules are comprised of just 20 building blocks, called *amino acids*. These, in turn, are bound together in long chains to form a wide range of protein types. How the amino acids are arranged dictates the protein's function and how it interacts with other cellular molecules.

Your DNA interacts with the real world through these proteins. The information stored in our DNA can only be used to make new proteins through a process called *protein synthesis*. There are no complex processors that interpret our DNA's information; in their most basic form, our genes only encode the sequence of amino acids that make a particular protein. Cellular processes take that information and make physical proteins that can interact with the rest of the human body. This means that, to activate or deactivate a gene, you would have to interfere with the process which converts DNA sequences into proteins. A gene is pretty much useless and doesn't affect our body, as long as it stays as pure information encoded in our DNA.

New proteins are made in two broad steps. First, the sequence of amino acids is read from a particular section of our DNA – called a gene – and then transcribed to another messenger protein. The start and end of these sections are well defined through special DNA blocks, helping the transcription process find a particular gene on our DNA.

We now know that there are approximately 22,000 unique genes encoded on our DNA, making these localization blocks quite important. If you lived in a city with 22,000 streets, you would need a pretty good GPS to help you navigate. Therefore, to make the protein generation process more efficient, we have these specialized sequences on our DNA that help direct transcription systems.

Once the information is read from our DNA, the messenger protein that copied a gene's amino acid sequence can leave the nucleus. It then travels to a molecular factory that lives inside almost all living cells, converting the messenger to the final protein.

What's critical to note about this process is that it can be controlled. Otherwise, all cells would behave the same, producing the same proteins over and over again. Some cells "know" to function as skin cells, while others act as liver cells. Living cells need a way to selectively produce only a subset of proteins specific to the type of a particular cell, to sustain the vast diversity of organs that make up the human body. This behavior can be regulated, not only through inherited procedures ingrained in our DNA but also through means that we can control ourselves.

The DNA is often portrayed as a long helix of nuclear molecules. In reality, it also has a complex shape and can coil onto itself. This twisting prevents messenger proteins from reaching some genes that are on coiled sections of the DNA. This way, the shape of our DNA dictates which genes are read, and ultimately the function of the cell. The genes are still there, but the messenger proteins can't reach them anymore.

This twisting allows cells to function differently depending on their location in the body, even if they have the same genetic composition. This is why the physical shape of the DNA is just as important as the raw information that is encoded on it. You can change how a cell works by shaping the DNA itself through knots made in places where you don't want a gene to be read. This form is usually ingrained in the DNA from the moment a cell is created and can't be changed by us directly. However, we do have other means at our disposal we can use to manipulate our DNA.

One other way to change which proteins are produced is to bind special molecules on the DNA itself. They are called *transcription factors* and can alter the rate at which specific proteins are made. These factors are also proteins, but they are made with the sole purpose of changing how other genes are read and synthesized from the DNA. The human DNA stores many genes, but only 3% of its length contains actual useful information. The rest is filled by so-called *regulatory sequences,* which help guide transcription factors to the place where they should bind.

There are likely thousands of transcription factors that control how proteins are produced. With over 22,000 unique genes, a big chunk of them must be dedicated to managing this regulatory process. Each gene can have a series of promoting or suppressing sequences that bind at the beginning of the gene strand. These unique sequences can either make the gene more or less likely to be converted into physical proteins, thus affecting the cell function and the general wellbeing of the body.

Typically, to read the amino acid pattern from a gene, special builder proteins (called polymerases) attach to the beginning of a gene and start assembling the messenger protein. However, a polymerase needs to find its way to the correct place on the DNA.

To help the polymerases find their way, some transcription factors can act as a sort of GPS for these proteins, directing them to the beginning of a gene. As a result, these transcription factors act as promoters, as they increase the rate at which proteins are made.

Genes can also have suppressing sequences that bind at the beginning of a DNA strand and which prevent the polymerase from functioning correctly. Genes usually have a mix of promoters and suppressors. Depending on which of these are activated, some proteins will be made in abundance, while others will be blocked completely.

This entire genetic dance can affect both microscopic processes that happen within the cell but also systematic changes that occur in the whole body. For example, some genes can start an entire chain of reactions that increases stress hormones production. A minuscule change that began in a single strand of DNA can make us feel more anxious and affects the entire body.

The same is true for acne as well. Some genes dictate how much sebum to produce, how sensitive the immune system is to foreign invaders, and which ingredients go into sebum. Transcription factors can act as promoters or suppressors of these acne genes. In the end, genes dictate how likely we are to breakout, and controlling them is critical in our fight against pimples.

The key to turning genes on and off is to control transcription factors that alter how genetic information is read from the DNA. The human body is usually self-regulating and has the right balance of promoting and suppressing factors.

For example, a unique gene encodes how to make a protein that can break down lactose (a type of sugar that we get from drinking milk). This gene senses if we've recently eaten dairy products and can increase the production of these unique proteins that can break down lactose. The lactose-gene can sense the body's nutritional state through a series of transcription factors that are affected by lactose and which can dial up or dial down the production of such proteins. Without this automated system, unnecessary proteins would continuously be made, even if no lactose is present in the body. This would waste precious nutrients and energy on stuff the human body doesn't need.

Transcription factors can also interact with one another. After all, they, too, are proteins that have to be encoded as unique genes, meaning they have their own set of suppressors and promoters. A protein can act as a promoter for another protein, which acts as a suppressor of a promoter of a suppressor... Argh!

If all of this sounds complicated, it's because it is. It took scientists decades of work to figure out all DNA sequences that help guide transcription factors and polymerase. Thankfully for us, we now live in a world where the entire genetic information from our DNA has been read. We now know the specific sequence of DNA molecules that make up all our genes. We might not know what all of them do, but we at least know their signature. This was a tremendous feat, considering that a single strand of DNA would measure 2 meters in length if uncoiled [47]. If you take the DNA from all cells in the human body – some several billion – and put them end to end, it would span the entire length from Earth to the Sun 70 times!

Acne is no different from any other bodily process; transcription factors influence most aspects that can lead to this disease. The genes that encode sebum production, inflammation, and cell turnover have their own set of transcription factors that act as promoters or suppressors. These genes can be turned on and off, thus influencing how likely we are to get pimples.

What's crucial to note about these transcription factors is that they are not only microscopic things that we have no control over. They can also be influenced by how we act and through what we eat. Ultimately, transcription factors sense the state in which we are in and monitor signals such as exhaustion, stress, nutrients level, age, etc. Genes can sense the environment we are in and how well we treat our bodies and act accordingly. To make these decisions, transcription factors need to have antennas in the body, including some that detect nutritional state.

Glucose and insulin can also act as transcription factors, thus helping the body maintain a perfect balance between energy usage and storage. For example, if we've recently eaten loads of carbs, the body has to store the excess energy as fat reserves. Similarly, if we've not eaten for some time and feel lightheaded, the body has to activate the conversion of fat back into glucose, thus giving cells energy. Genes and gene transcription factors regulate these processes. Such factors sense whether we have sufficient glucose in the bloodstream and, if not, turn on the process that converts fat reserves back into glucose [48].

*

One specific class of transcription factors that control fat reserves is *Sterol regulatory element-binding proteins* (SREBPs) — considered the primary regulators of lipid production and synthesis in the human body. There are multiple versions of transcription factors that fall in the SREBP group. Some manage global lipid production, while others control fatty acid creation. These factors are critical in cell growth and nutrition, as they support the production of raw material needed to repair existing cells or create new ones.

Although they have mostly beneficial effects, overly activated SREBPs have also been found to negatively affect the body, mainly through their involvement with cancer, diabetes, and obesity [49]. If SREBPs produce too many lipids, they can cause excessive fat to accumulate in cells, leading to so-called *lipotoxicity*. As a result, cells can become stressed, eventually leading to cellular dysfunction and death.

Seeing as sebum is comprised predominately of fat molecules [26], it's natural to assume that SREBPs also control sebum production. Indeed, that is what recent experimental data suggests. It was found that SREBPs manage not only the rate at which sebum flows [50] but also its composition. When activated, SREBPs increase the rate at which skin cells produce sebum, potentially boosting the chances of clogs forming in skin pores.

SREBPs don't control only the production of sebum but also its composition. As it turns out, the over-activation of SREBPs increases the output of monosaturated fats, which are thicker than normal sebum. Oleic acid, for example, is one type of monosaturated fat, and it is twice as thick as squalene (a major component of sebum) [51] [52]. It is over-produced in skin cells with stimulated SREBPs factors [53]. If these thick substances are produced in abundance, they will get mixed with the other sebum ingredients to make the entire mixture more viscous. If this happens, pore blockages are more likely, as thick and sticky sebum will tend to clog our pores more often.

Thicker sebum does not promote only pore blockages but also bacterial growth and inflammation. Oleic acid, which is more viscous than normal sebum, increases the adhesion of bacteria to the skin – including the acne-promoting bacteria. If more oleic acid gets mixed in with sebum, it will create a sticky protective film that adheres to our skin's outer layer in which bacteria can multiply freely [54]. In these conditions, more bacteria will be released in our skin when pimples form, causing a worse inflammatory response. More so, oleic acid directly stimulates the production of pro-inflammatory proteins, making the immune system more sensitive to the presence of bacteria [55].

Overall, the SREBP group of transcription factors is a major aggravator of acne – they promote sebum production and composition changes, enhance bacterial growth, and increase inflammation.

Although SREBPs are important actors for acne, they can be controlled. Evidence suggests that by managing the signals that activate SREBPs, we can also suppress the over-production of lipids and sebum, thereby reducing the risk of developing acne. This brings us back to the glucose and insulin discussed earlier in this chapter. It is now believed that both insulin and glucose cause an entire cascade of transcription factor changes, ultimately leading to overly stimulated SREBPs and an increased risk of acne.

Tests performed on isolated skin cells found that low doses of insulin are relatively harmless, while high doses of insulin cause increased production of specific proteins in the SREBP family. When stimulated with insulin, sebum glands produce three times more sebum compared to normal [50]. Similar results were found for hormones that mimick insulin – aptly named *insulin-like growth factors.*

Experiments show that high glycemic foods can cause acne by increasing insulin production, thus affecting the balance of SREBPs transcription factors. This link between insulin and SREBPs also explains why acne patients who eliminate fast carbs from their diet see an improvement in pimple count. Experiments have shown that people who eliminate foods that active SREBPs will have smaller sebum-producing glands and improved acne scores [45].

Overall, the connection between fast carbs and acne is one of the strongest that we know for this disease. Epidemiological studies have shown that acne patients tend to eat more carbs and drink more sugary beverages than average. Interventional studies demonstrated that acne improves in patients who eliminate high-glycemic foods from their diet. And in-vitro tests found a plausible explanation of this effect by studying the interaction between insulin and SREBP transcription factors. Overall, although there is a genetic component to acne, these genes can be controlled. Our DNA doesn't shape who we are; instead, we shape our DNA through what we eat and how we interact with the environment.

SREBPs are not the only transcription factors that can affect acne, far from it. Sebum is one part of the equation, but we've yet to look at inflammation, skin cell turnover, or oxidation. More so, insulin is not the only molecule that affects SREBPs; many other dietary factors can influence lipid production and other secondary processes that promote acne.

As mentioned previously, the human body is self-regulating. It "knows" when to turn on and off specific metabolic processes to keep an optimal balance. In this chapter, we've looked at one very small part in the series of transcription factors that sense nutritional state, but the body can detect other aspects, including our age. As we go from birth into adulthood, our bodies go through several transformations that help us grow in size, accentuate our sex, and make us smarter. These changes are also governed by our genes and by transcription factors.

Because lipids are an essential part when building new cells, it's reasonable to assume that we would need to make more of this stuff at the stages of our life when we need to grow and create new cells. For this reason, it is now believed that lipid and sebum production is heavily constrained by the same governors that control human growth in childhood and adolescence.

However, just like general lipid production, the growth-sensing transcription factors can also be tricked by our diet, leading to complications that negatively affect our health and our skin. By providing our bodies with artificial signals that mimic body growth, we trick our cells into producing more sebum than they should. When we do this, we're not actually growing, but our bodies think we are. We will look at how and why this happens in the next chapter.

CHAPTER SUMMARY

- Several epidemiological studies have shown that people who eat lots of sugars or carb-rich foods have an increased risk of developing acne.

- Results from clinical trials have also shown that acne patients who follow a low-glycemic diet will develop fewer pimples.

- Insulin is a hormone that is released in high quantities when eating sugars or fast carbs.

- Genes control how cells function, but they can be turned on and off by so-called transcription factors.

- One set of transcription factors, called SREBPs, act as master regulators of lipid production, also controlling sebum composition and flow rate.

- Insulin acts as a promoter of SREBPs, driving compositional changes to sebum, making it stickier and more prone to cause pore blockages and acne. This interaction between insulin and sebum explains why people on a high-carb diet tend to develop more acne.

MEAT

Meat is a staple food in nearly every Western country, being present in almost all meals. For most, vegetables are considered a side dish, and no meal is complete without some meat. There is a growing number of vegans and vegetarians in Western nations, but regular meat-eaters still form the majority [56]. As a result, 80% of current agricultural land is dedicated to raising livestock, even if meat supplies only 20% of the world's calories [57]. If all nations switched to an average American diet, there wouldn't be enough land on Earth to feed everyone, not even if we convert all the desserts and tropical forests into farmlands, and we would live in floating cities [57].

Meat is such a popular food item because it's renowned for being rich in protein (and because steak tastes great). Although protein is usually considered the most important nutrient you can get in your diet, most people don't understand why it is essential and what the alternatives are. Even the word "protein" stems from the Greek word *Proteios,* which translates as "of prime importance." This craze in protein is widespread among athletes, where protein shakes are promoted to improve physical performance, endurance and build muscle. Meat is considered the best source of protein, and no athlete should go a meal without it.

However, after reading through the previous chapter, you likely have an intuition that this is not necessarily true. Our body uses protein for many different functions, including converting the information from our DNA into useful products. This is true for all living creatures — be it plants, insects, fish, or mammals. Proteins and amino acids are critical to life, which is why they are also present in nearly everything we eat. You would have to try really hard *not* to get enough protein from your diet by eating only sugar and tree bark. Yet, if proteins are present in almost everything we eat, then why do we have the myth that only meat contains "good" protein sources?

When people recommend including more protein in our diet, they really refer to the building blocks of these molecules – the amino acids. Every living creature can create all the protein it needs from scratch. We only need the genetic information stored in our DNA and the raw amino acids we normally get from our diet.

As mentioned in the previous chapter, to make protein, the genetic sequence stored on a particular gene is first copied onto a temporary messenger protein, which then travels out of the nucleus to the protein factory. Here, amino acids are stitched together in the correct sequence to form the final protein structure.

If you remember from basic biology lessons, the DNA is comprised of just four molecules arranged in pairs: guanine, adenine, cytosine, and thymine; often shortened as G, A, C, and T. These are part of the nucleotides family of organic molecules. A sequence of three such molecules defines which amino acid should bind at that specific site. For example, if in a DNA sequence you find the nucleotides CTC-CAG-GCT, this tells you that you should first assemble a leucine amino-acid, followed by glutamine, and then cap it off with alanine. At the end of a protein sequence, a unique series of nucleotides tell the protein factory to stop assembly and release the final product. To make this sequence complete, we can add these terminal nucleotides and encode our protein as CTC-CAG-GCT-TAA. There, we've just made our first protein.

Obviously, real-world proteins are much more complex than this. The longest protein chain that we know is made of 34,350 amino acids and is aptly named Titin (derived from *Titans,* the ancient Greek gods) [58]. Our bodies use this protein to build muscle fibers, giving them their elasticity. No wonder muscles are so hungry for amino acids.

Although most proteins have a complex shape and structure, the basic principle of building them is still the same. Cells use raw building blocks in the form of amino acids and assemble the final protein structure using the sequence defined in a gene. Because of this, we only need to eat the raw amino acids; Mother Nature does the rest. We can break down the protein that we eat (and the ones in our cells as well; more on that later) to release and store amino acids.

We can make some of the amino acids ourselves from scratch. Others, we can only get from our diet. The human body has evolved this way because making amino acids requires considerable amounts of energy. Why waste excess energy making amino acids from scratch if we can get enough from our diet? This is the reason why humans and most animals have lost the ability to synthesize certain amino acids that we usually get enough from what we eat. This also means that humans, to be healthy, need to eat a sufficiently varied diet to ensure we get enough of these nutrients that we can't make ourselves.

The amino acids that we can't produce are called *essential* amino acids and are predominantly made in plants. Most animals can't make these essential nutrients either, but they do eat a plant-based diet that contains them. Throughout the life of animals, their meat accumulates all essential amino acids, which are passed down to us once we eat them.

This is the reason why some consider meat protein sources superior. Animals can't make essential amino acids either, but they do eat a plant-based diet (or eat other animals that consume plants), which contains these nutrients. Thus, they accumulate nutrients throughout their life, providing us with a concentrated meal of proteins and amino acids.

Despite all of this, there's no reason why we can't cut the middle man and get all our nutrients from plants ourselves. It's the way the human body has evolved to do, and tipping this balance point can cause serious health problems. Yet, this type of imbalance is common – and often recommended – as part of a Western diet.

We now obsess over getting enough protein in our diet from animal sources. Currently, the average American consumes twice as much protein as the recommended daily dose – most of it coming from animal sources [59] [60]. Because we consume more protein than what our bodies evolved to support, we've started developing more human-made diseases, including some forms of cancer and potentially acne as well.

Animal protein is currently being studied for its ability to be a cancer tumor accelerant. In-vitro cells exposed to aflatoxin – a potent carcinogen – showed substantial tumor growth on cells extracted from lab mice fed a diet based on animal protein. However, if the same carcinogen was applied to cells collected from rats on a low-protein diet, the tumor-promoting enzyme activity was reduced by 76% [61].

Similar studies have shown that tumor precursor cells grow in significantly higher quantities in the liver when following a diet rich in protein. Animals fed a high-casein diet (a protein found predominantly in milk and dairy products) had four times the tumor growth activity compared to the low-casein diet [62].

Because of these findings, animal protein is currently being investigated as a possible carcinogen for liver cancer. Some medical researchers now recommend following a low protein diet (under 10% of daily calory intake) to protect against these forms of cancer [63].

How does all of this tie in with acne? The same cancer-promoting processes, which are overly stimulated in a protein-rich diet, also activate several transcription factors that can lead to acne.

So far, we've learned of one class of transcription factors that play an important role in acne growth, namely SREBPs. They control sebum production and its composition. SREBPs are also highly stimulated by insulin and glucose, so they are sensitive to foods with lots of sugars and fast carbs.

We've also seen that transcription factors interact with one another, creating a complex cascade of cell changes that can either dial-up or dial-down the production of proteins. SREBPs are terminal transcription factors, but what happens before is just as important. Recent evidence suggests that other genes can mediate SREBP activity, paving the way for more ways to fight acne. As we'll see later on, it seems that animal protein can interfere with these cellular processes that drive sebum production, making us more prone to breaking out.

Lipids are used in a wide range of cellular functions and are vital building blocks when creating new cells. The largest quantity of lipids is used to make the outer membrane of new cells, meaning you can't grow organs without significant amounts of lipids. Because of this, during certain stages of our life, we must produce sufficient scaffolding material to support the creation of new cells – particularly during childhood and puberty. During this period, the body must ramp up lipid production to support the new growth which happens throughout our body.

SREBPs support this process as they can drive up lipid production during childhood to provide enough raw material for new cells. But it only makes sense to turn on the factors if we're eating enough nutrients to support this new growth. As a result, SREBPs don't act independently. They have overseers that sense the body's nutritional state and dictate when SREBPs should dial-up lipid and sebum production. These overseers are also transcription factors, but they are sensitive to other nutrients besides glucose and insulin. Notably, the growth regulators have antennas for growth signals (in the form of specific hormones) and amino acids that can come in abundance from meat. Next, we will look at how excessive proteins can fool these central governors into dialing up sebum production.

The master regulator of growth

Easter Island has been on my travel bucket list for a long time, but unfortunately, it's also one of the most remote places you can visit. The island measures only 164 km^2, which is roughly the same size as Liechtenstein. It is officially part of the territory of Chile, but the distance between the capital of Chile and Easter Island measures just over 3,700 Km, or about the same distance from Madrid to Moscow. From where I live, a flight to Easter Island takes 57 hours, has four stops, and costs as much as a small car. Thankfully, my travel bucket list is quite long, so I have plenty of time to save up my money and energy.

This region is renowned for its cultural heritage, which is quite unique compared to anything you've seen before, being helped by the island's remoteness. Easter Island is quite famous for its giant human-like statues, weighing up to 80 tonnes, carved from a single block of stone. Under 8,000 inhabitants live permanently on this island, and the first colonists are estimated to have arrived as early as 300 AD. Who would have thought that, in this small and remote island, we would discover a molecule many consider to be the fountain of youth and which is currently investigated for its cancer-fighting ability.

In 1972, a group of researchers based on Easter Island discovered an unknown anti-microbial substance extracted from bacteria that naturally grows in the region. Subsequent studies showed that this substance prevents the growth of certain fungi and can suppress the immune system in more complex organisms [64]. Because of these effects, this product was later approved by the FDA to be used following organ transplants to prevent the receiving body from rejecting the new organ. This drug was named rapamycin, after the region in which it was discovered (Easter Island is also named Rapa Nui).

Rapamycin has been the center point of numerous experiments since then, as it was eventually found to suppress cell growth in almost all living organisms, including fruit flies, bacteria, fungi, plants, and even mammals [64]. Because rapamycin has immunosuppressant properties, it was initially thought that it would promote cancer growth, as it dampens the body's system that kills new tumor cells. However, when this molecule was tested on various cancers, it was found to have the opposite effect – it inhibits the growth of several cancers found in humans [65]. Currently, rapamycin analogs are widely used in cancer therapy [66].

Another surprising effect of rapamycin is that it can prolong life in some organisms. This is remarkable considering that this drug suppresses the immune system and new cell growth, making organisms more sensitive to infection and other transmissible diseases. However, when tested, rapamycin was found to increase the lifespan of a wide range of living creatures, from yeast to mammals.

In 2009, it was found that mice who were treated with this drug had a prolonged life, living 9% to 14% more than average [67]. Although we've previously observed this effect in more primitive life forms (such as fruit flies [68]), this was the first evidence to suggest that the longevity-promoting effect of rapamycin can also be applied to mammals and potentially humans as well. Since 2009, other studies have confirmed this positive effect on mice [69], hence why rapamycin has gained its reputation as the "fountain of youth."

However, because rapamycin also suppresses the immune system, it's too risky to verify if the same effects apply to humans as well. The mice from these studies lived in sanitary and controlled conditions, devoid of real-life viruses and bacteria that can degrade health. Although rapamycin might prolong cell life in ideal conditions, it also opens the door for other diseases to enter. We would probably die from infectious diseases long before we would reap the benefits of rapamycin. It's not exactly wise to take rapamycin as a supplement if you plan on living outside of a sanitary bubble. To reap these health benefits, we would need to isolate the longevity-promoting effects of rapamycin without the complications to the immune system.

The initial discovery that propelled our understanding of aging was made when scientists found that rapamycin does not directly promote longevity and tumor suppression. Instead, it acts through another protein, aptly named *target of rapamycin*. In turn, this protein was found in a wide range of species, ranging from yeast up to humans. These molecules have a unique signature in mammals, hence why they were further characterized as *mammalian target of rapamycin* (mTOR). In humans, mTOR forms a symbiotic union with at least two other proteins, creating unique groups of proteins (or protein complexes) that serve various roles in our bodies.

Since the discovery of mTOR, we now know that this protein, alongside its complexes, is responsible for managing cell growth and division in mammals and humans. mTOR is the true "fountain of youth," while rapamycin is just one way we can manipulate it.

mTOR is the central regulator of cell growth and multiplication in most living creatures. It helps ensure that, when needed, the organism can create new cells to support either organ reparation or the expansion of existing organs. Because mTOR is a protein like any other (meaning it is encoded in a gene and has unique transcription factors), it can be either turned on or turned off by various factors. If not kept in an optimal state, the body can be put out of balance, leading to diseases that are dependent on excessive cell growth.

Acne is also a disease that is primarily driven by excess growth. Sebum and skin cell overproduction can create pore clogs, while excessive immune cells can make the skin more sensitive to inflammation. Thus, mTOR is now also believed to influence acne by either promoting or repressing functions that depend on growth, making us more prone to breaking out.

mTOR itself does not directly cause cell multiplication. Instead, it ensures that these processes happen correctly and safely. When new cells need to be created, sufficient energy and raw building material need to be present in the body. mTOR ensures that these two preconditions are met before allowing further body growth.

mTOR needs to receive two broad signals before it gives the green light to the cell multiplication process. First, a growth signal must be emitted somewhere in the body, instructing cells to start the multiplication process. Secondly, mTOR also listens for the body's nutritional state, being tuned to detect if we have sufficient building blocks to create new cells.

Most of the growth that we observe happens from childhood to early adulthood. In this period, growth signals are emitted, usually in the form of insulin or hormones that mimic insulin (more on this later). In this period, we grow significantly in height and mass, and mTOR partially supports this process. In the growth stages of our life, special hormones are secreted, which tell various organs that they should develop to maturity. mTOR listens to these hormones and ensures cell multiplication happens as expected.

Although most of the visible growth happens in childhood, some organs and systems continue to regenerate cells throughout our lives. For example, red blood cells must continuously be created to support good organ oxygenation. mTOR governs the creation of new red blood cells when sufficient nutrients are present (particularly iron), ensuring normal bodily function [70]. For this reason, mTOR responds to other growth signals besides the ones secreted during childhood. Notably, insulin and glucose are secreted throughout our life and help drive new cell growth and regeneration [71].

Besides growth hormones, cells also need sufficient nutrients and scaffolding material to multiplicate correctly. mTOR has antennas for nutrients as well, thus ensuring the body has enough building blocks before attempting to create new cells. These nutrient probes respond to a wide range of molecules, but the most important classes are amino acids and certain fats. Interestingly, not all amino acids activate mTOR the same way. Particularly, *leucine* (an amino acid predominantly found in dairy products) and *arginine* (an amino acid abundant in meat) have a higher effect on mTOR compared to other molecules in this group [72].

mTOR is the convergence point of many different food groups, which is why it's so easily abused by our diet. A typical Western meal contains all the ingredients necessary to over stimulate mTOR, namely insulin (from sugary beverages and fast carbs), proteins, and fat (from meat sources).

Why is this a bad thing? After all, mTOR should coordinate with the rest of the body to ensure the correct functioning of critical processes that depend on cell division. Why would too many nutrients be harmful to us, and how does this affect our skin?

The answer to this lies partly with how cells manage waste and how mTOR helps clean this waste. If a parent cell doesn't have sufficient amino acids to function correctly, mTOR boosts the breaking down of existing proteins into their constituents. This way, a cell can make all the necessary building blocks needed for growth, essentially recycling old and discarded proteins.

The first proteins to be recycled are usually the ones created in normal cellular processes but which have served their purpose and are no longer useful. If left unattended, discarded proteins continue to build up in cells, eventually leading to cell damage and death. Even in your own house, if you don't take out the trash for long enough, garbage will start to build all around you, creating the perfect breeding grounds for bacteria, fungi, and other harmful pathogens. Living in filth for long enough will only deteriorate your health. The same is true for all living cells in our bodies. They, too, create waste that needs to be periodically taken out not to damage the cell itself.

Because of this, it's essential to break down discarded proteins periodically to ensure cellular trash doesn't accumulate to the point that it starts to harm cells. mTOR helps direct this cleanup through a process called autophagy.

If mTOR senses that there aren't enough amino acids in a cell, it promotes autophagy to break down waste proteins into the raw amino acids, thus discarding cells of their trash. This process has been found to decrease cancer tumor growth [73] [74], protect against neurodegenerative diseases [75] [76], prevent infectious diseases [77] [78], and generally increase lifespan [79].

It may seem counter-intuitive that, by starving yourself, you can live longer. But this seems to be the case, at least up to a certain point. On nutrient restriction, cells don't actually starve; they just consume waste products. But even this can last only for so long. Eventually, cells do run out of trash to break down, so an optimal balance must be kept.

We go through this cleanup process each time we go between meals. For most modern humans, this corresponds to nighttime when we are asleep, and we don't consume any food. During this period, glucose and insulin levels are at their lowest, allowing mTOR to function fully.

However, because most of us live on diets that over-stimulate mTOR, the fasting that we go through each night doesn't seem to be enough anymore to prevent certain diseases. The human body has evolved to go through long periods without food while it hunts and gathers fresh food to eat. mTOR is tuned to work in these stretches of intermittent fasting, which unfortunately don't exist anymore in modern times. When we're hungry, we take a snack, thus preventing mTOR from breaking down cellular waste.

Furthermore, mTOR directly stimulates the production of new proteins, compounding the problem even more [80]. When we overindulge, it tells mTOR to create new proteins instead of breaking down old ones, adding to the trash that already existent in cells.

These observations have spun new diets that promote calorie restriction to improve longevity and general health. They go under the name *intermittent fasting diets* and are becoming increasingly popular. By restricting the hours we eat, we give mTOR more time to recycle cell waste, thus improving our health.

Besides its involvement with protein creation and recycling, mTOR also mediates lipid production. To create new cells, the body needs lipids to build the outer membrane, hence why mTOR must ensure sufficient fat molecules are present before starting the multiplication process. When mTOR is activated, an entire cascade of in-cell changes is initiated, leading to more fatty molecules being made. Because of this, it should come as no surprise that mTOR also controls the master regulators of lipid and sebum, namely the SREBPs transcription factors [81].

In-vitro tests showed that SREBP activation is dependent upon mTOR signaling. Although SREBPs have their own set of antennas that sense the environment and dictate when to produce lipids, these antennas only work if mTOR is in an activated state [81]. If you suppress mTOR, then you also cut the ties between SREBP and the environment, thus preventing lipid and sebum production.

The sebum factory doesn't depend only on the signal which directly activates SREBPs, but also on the factors that stimulate mTOR. Indeed, it was found that if you only suppress mTOR, you also decrease the rate at which sebum is made [82]. Furthermore, it was found that, by switching mTOR off, we also prevent some other related factors which give rise to acne, such as sebum compositional changes and bacterial growth [82].

In the previous chapter, we saw that sugars heavily influence sebum glands. People that undergo a low-sugar diet will improve their acne condition as their sebum production decreases while the sebum itself becomes less sticky and less prone to blockages [45]. Previously, we thought that this effect is only due to the SREBP family of transcription factors, as they are susceptible to high glycemic loads in our blood. Now, we can see that sugars don't affect only the SREBPs but also mTOR, further amplifying the acne-inducing effect. Sugar stimulates the production of sebum by activating both SREBPs and mTOR. Other food groups have this snowball effect as well, and we will explore them more throughout this book.

mTOR also plays an essential role in managing the immune system. This happens both at a local level, by mediating the inflammation response to a site of injury; and globally in the entire body, by stimulating the whole immune system to produce white blood cells that can fight infection and foreign pathogens. Both are important factors when managing acne, but arguably local inflammation needs special attention. Pimples form when the skin becomes inflamed, so any factors that amplify this effect can exacerbate acne.

Previous research has shown that mTOR stimulates both T cell production (a type of white blood cell essential to the immune system) and the creation of pro-inflammatory proteins [83]. When the body creates new T cells, they are initially put in a state of dormancy to reduce the metabolic cost of keeping them alive. This process is similar to how bears hibernate during the winter; they transition to a state of minimal activity to make sure nutrients last all winter. When an infection does occur, T cells move into an activated state and start fighting off foreign pathogens and cancer cells. However, because being in an activated state is expensive to the body, if T cells lack appropriate energy and nutrients reserves, they simply die off.

To prevent immune cells from dying prematurely from a lack of nutrients, mTOR mediates T cell activity by sensing the cell's nutrients state before providing the all-clear signal for cells to turn on and start fighting infection [83]. This process is crucial in preventing the over-use of nutrients by the immune system and excessive T cell death.

If we over-activate mTOR, too many T cells can move out of hibernation. Even if there are sufficient nutrients to sustain this process, this can still lead to health complications. Particularly, if the immune system is too active, it can start attacking the host body through what we now call auto-immune diseases. This is why mTOR regulation is currently being investigated as a possible treatment for this class of diseases [84].

Similarly, the same imbalance in T cell activity is now also thought to be involved with acne formation, as T cell infiltrates are found in early acne lesions [85]. If mTOR is put into a state of overdrive, it makes the skin more sensitive to foreign invaders (such as when acne-promoting bacteria infiltrates the skin), increasing inflammation and making us more likely to break out.

Besides its involvement with the immune system, mTOR was also found to stimulate the production of pro-inflammatory proteins in the skin. When a foreign pathogen is detected by skin cells (like when you injure your skin and bacteria gets infiltrated), the cells near the lesion produce signaling proteins that direct immune-system cells to the affected region. These proteins cause the blood vessels to open up, thus increasing blood flow, helping with recovery. However, this opening up of the blood vessels also causes local inflammation in the skin.

The same inflammatory response likewise leads to the dreaded pimples if too many pro-inflammatory proteins are released. Recent experiments have shown that skin cells release more of these inflammatory proteins when local mTOR is activated [86]. When rapamycin was administered to skin cells exposed to irritants, pro-inflammatory protein production decreased to less than a third of the baseline sample. This insight shows yet another critical function of mTOR when relating to acne. When pimples form, mTOR directs the skin to be more sensitive to bacteria, worsening inflammation and making our breakout even worse.

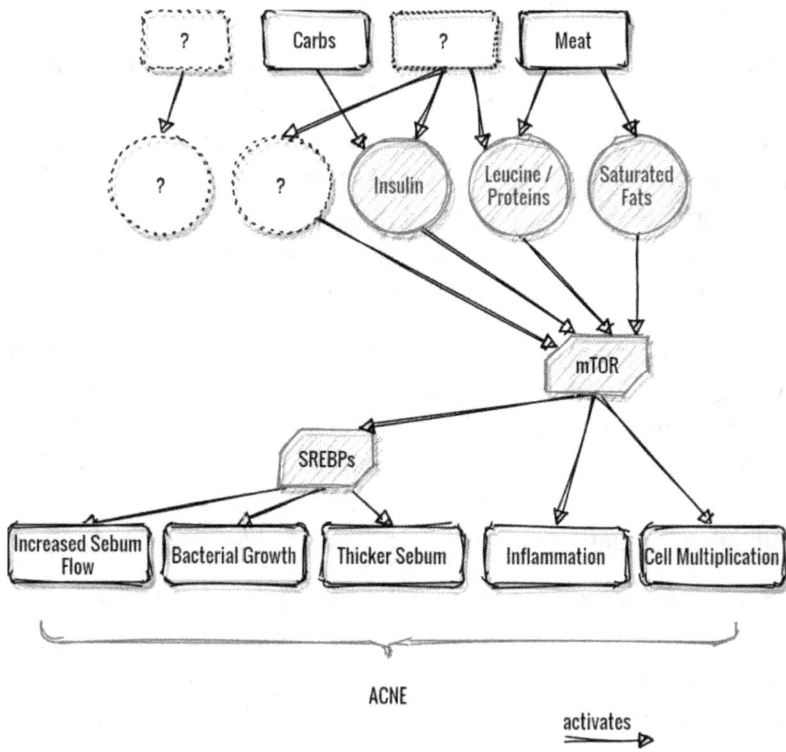

Figure 2 - Effects of meat and sugars on mTOR

As you can see, mTOR is the convergence point of a lot of different factors that eventually lead to acne. On the one hand, mTOR drives sebum production and compositional changes by stimulating SREBPs. It promotes skin cell multiplication, providing material for pore clogs. Lastly, mTOR accelerates local inflammation, making it more likely for pimples to form once bacteria infiltrate the skin.

Because of all these factors, managing mTOR is proven to be crucial in preventing acne. Studies that compare the diets of acne patients with that of clear-skin individuals generally find that eating foods with low mTOR affinity is protective against this disease. For example, one study found that a vegan diet is potentially beneficial to our skin. If you follow this diet, your risk of developing pimples drops to half compared to the general population [87].

Although following a vegan diet was found to be protective in general, we now know that only some food items should be avoided if we want to keep our skin clear.

Leucine is an amino acid that is abundantly found in some animal-derived foods, especially in meat and milk. It is also one amino acid that heavily simulates mTOR, making us more likely to develop pimples. These insights were found while studying athletes that regularly consume protein shakes containing concentrated forms of leucine. Athletes that start protein supplementation to improve psychical performance develop acne after this diet change [88]. This is because the most common protein supplement is whey protein, which is derived from leucine-rich milk. Although other food items contain leucine, protein supplements tend to be highly concentrated and deliver excessive doses of amino acids.

Besides milk and whey protein, other animal food sources (and meat in particular) also tend to be rich in protein, which can activate mTOR. For example, to get the same amount of leucine from 100 g of steak, you would have to eat 4.2 kg of white cabbage or 100 apples [82]. Arginine (another potent mTOR activator) is also found abundantly in animal products. You would have to eat 30 times more sweet potatoes to get the same amount of arginine as a single serving of turkey breast [89] [90].

The fact that meat is highly concentrated in amino acids that stimulate mTOR is the reason why this food group can be problematic to our skin. By excessively eating meat, we give a high dose of amino acids to our cells, instructing them to grow and multiply when they really shouldn't. In turn, this causes excessive lipid (and sebum) production, increased turnover for skin cells, and excessive inflammation, all of which can make us more likely to breakout.

It should be noted that an underactive mTOR can be just as damaging. Insufficient nutrition during early childhood can lead to stunted growth [91], while an underactive mTOR during adulthood can cause muscle atrophy [92]. However, in Western countries, it's much more likely to find people with an overactivated mTOR due to an over-abundance of protein, sugars, and fats from our diet. Some speculate that the increase in human-made diseases in developed nations is due in part to mTOR, leading to an unexpected decrease in life expectancy in certain countries that follow diets with a high mTOR affinity (particularly the USA) [93].

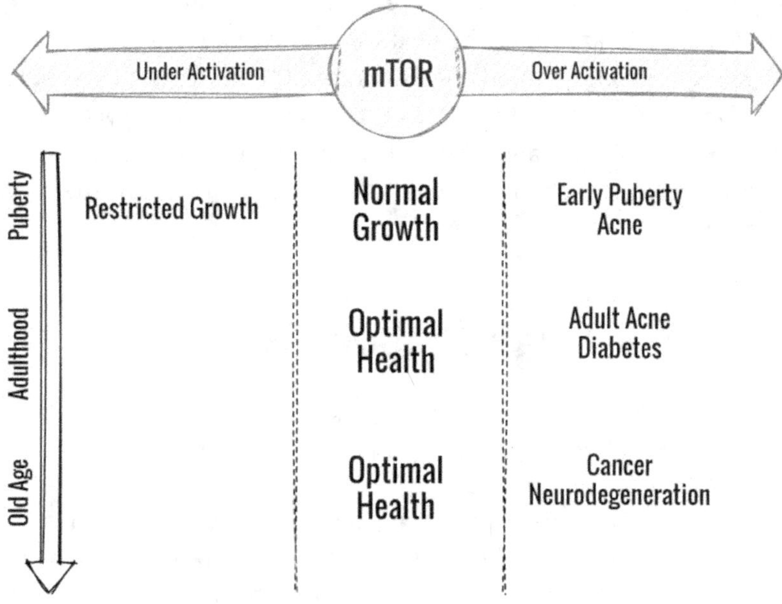

Figure 3 - Effects of over or underactivation of mTOR

Although mTOR's implications in modern diseases – such as cancer or diabetes – are still being explored, most researchers in the field of dermatology agree that acne is primarily an mTOR-driven disease [82]. Still, this is far from enough to explain all possible causes of acne. We still have to explain why acne is more common during adolescence and why some people break out during stressful life events. mTOR is not the only governor of acne, and protein and sugars are not the only signals to mTOR. More so, recent evidence has uncovered a new set of transcription factors, which potentially manage mTOR, SREBPs, and other components that can lead to acne. Interestingly, these factors are also controlled by diet, but in a way that is the exact opposite to how mTOR operates.

During periods of prosperity, mTOR enables the body to grow and flourish. However, when times are tough, the body needs a separate governor that must direct cells to conserve nutrients to make sure we make it to the next meal. Although relatively few of us still go through periods of starvation, the systems that ensure survival are still with us from our ancestors. The same process that provided our endurance in prehistoric times might also prove crucial in our fight against acne. We will look at how in the next chapter.

CHAPTER SUMMARY

- mTOR is a protein that is regarded as the master regulator of cellular growth and division.

- mTOR governs protein production, promotes lipid synthesis, and mediates the SREBPs transcription factors. Because of this, mTOR is a central convergence point for acne, as it manages sebum production, inflammation, and skin cell multiplication.

- Meat and sugars over-stimulate mTOR, leading to an entire cascade of body changes that can cause acne.

- A vegan diet was found to be protective against acne, as it limits the intake of amino acids that were found to activate mTOR. Similarly, eating foods rich in proteins – such as meat or protein shakes – was found to aggravate acne.

DAIRY

Isn't it strange that humans are the only known species who will regularly consume milk after weaning? Yes, a cat will happily drink milk if offered, but it's still not something we naturally see in the wild. Milk has evolved to provide an optimal set of nutrients to a newborn baby – antibodies, protein, lactose, and growth factors – but we are actively consuming it well into our adulthood. Frequently drinking a cocktail of growth hormones, excessive proteins, and antibodies meant for a completely different species is likely not a very good idea. This, in the context where previous research has already linked regular consumption of dairy products with an increased risk of Parkinson's [94] [95], prostate cancer [96], type 1 diabetes [97], and the most well-known associations of all: heart disease [98] [99] [100] [101].

Although scientific research tends to sway on putting dairy products on the do-not-consume list, milk is still generally promoted as a healthy drink. Most people have seen milk commercials touting milk's health benefits for our bones due to it being rich in calcium. However, scientific research shows quite the opposite. High calcium intake does little to reduce the risk of fractures [102] [103]. More so, in some age groups, milk consumption is associated with brittle bones [104]. This contrarian observation is likely from the high protein concentration of milk, which has been found to breakdown bones by promoting the excretion of calcium [105].

Given that regular consumption of dairy products has been tied to numerous health risks and that high-calcium diets do little for bone health, why are we still recommending this food group as part of a "balanced and healthy diet"? The FDA still has dairy products on the list of recommended foods schoolchildren should eat [106], contradicting all the research done up until his point.

The answer to this is quite simple: the Dairy Industry generates 442 billion dollars in revenue yearly [107], which is more than the entire GDP of Austria [108]. And, as with any profitable business, the Dairy Industry takes steps to protect this cash cow. These include, but are not limited to, advertisement and funding research to promote the "health" benefits of this product.

We're already starting to see signs that sustaining a health-promoting industry on advertisement alone is not enough. For example, the US saw a reduction in the consumption of dairy products by around 40% from 1970 to 2013. To counteract the recent damaging scientific reports, the Dairy Industry has taken to "neutralizing the negative image of milkfat by regulators and medical professionals" [109]. Why make a product healthier when it's enough just to make it look so?

Plenty of books have been written on the subject of data manipulation and how to sway scientific results in your favor. My personal favorite is *How to Lie with statistics*, by Darrell Huff. It's not the most comprehensive on the subject, but it's a great introduction to anyone new to statistics. From this book, you'll see that there are a lot of different ways to change the interpretations of hard numbers to get the results you are after. Numbers don't lie, but you can still devise experiments such that a favorable outcome is pretty much guaranteed.

One such recent study proposed to summarize 29 other research papers linking dairy to various health effects. The paper concluded that "neutral associations of total, high and low-fat dairy, milk and yogurt with risk of all-cause mortality, [Congenital heart defect] and [Cardiovascular disease]" and "a possible role of fermented dairy was found in [Cardiovascular disease] prevention" [110]. This analysis found not only that dairy is neutral for heart disease, but it might also be protective if we consume certain fermented products, such as yogurt. These results go against most other studies on this topic that show the exact opposite.

If you read through the research paper, a first red flag will appear once you reach the funding section. Anyone can write a scientific paper in whatever format they want, but to be peer-reviewed and published in a respectable journal, you usually have to be transparent about who is paying for the respective experiment. Because of this, research papers have a special section at the end dedicated to disclosing the funding source and any other conflicts of interest. The same is true for this specific paper as well; if you look at the bottom, you'll notice that it was funded by the "Global Dairy Platform, Dairy Research Institute, and Dairy Australia." In other words, the Dairy Industry financed research that uncovered that dairy has no adverse effects on the heart and can be protective in specific scenarios. That's one big coincidence.

This doesn't mean that the research itself is invalid, but that we have to be especially critical when analyzing such papers. Meta-analysis can be more easily manipulated than other types of experiments, as you can simply cherry-pick which studies you want to be included in your findings. More so, you can also re-interpret the findings of the analyzed research papers to make the conclusions more in line with your narrative.

The Dairy Industry is notorious for pulling these kinds of stunts, even partnering with governments to fund research favorable to them. In Canada, for example, the Dairy Industry partnered with the federal government to finance the Dairy Research Cluster, with the primary objective of researching the nutritional benefits of milk and milk-derived products. In 2016, there were 23 active research projects in this organization, with more than 100 active scientists [111].

A professor in the department of surgical sciences at Uppsala University in Sweden was quoted saying, "Most likely, those who select projects to be funded [...] will possibly try to select projects that express a wish to present dairy in a positive way" [111]. In other words, this union will likely fund only research that has a high chance of putting dairy in a good light. As expected, industry-funded research has a high success rate for the sponsor, whereby 93% of scientific papers published by a particular food industry had positive results [111].

Because of these conflicts of interest, finding credible research on the health effects of dairy products (including acne) can be problematic. The confusion created by industry-sponsored research is widespread, hence why milk is still highly regarded as a health-promoting drink.

On the topic of acne, because milk is a cocktail that promotes growth for young offsprings, we would expect to be some interaction between this food group and our body's master regulator of growth, namely mTOR. Indeed, this is what one group of researchers sought to find out by studying the association between regular milk consumption and acne.

The study itself began in 2000 when the researchers asked adolescents aged 15 to 16 to fill out a form describing various aspects of their lifestyle. This form also included questions on the general diet, including dairy product consumption, such as skimmed or full-fat milk. A total of 3811 students participated in this study.

Four years later, in 2004, the same group of children, now aged 18 to 19, were asked to assess their acne's severity by recollecting the number of pimples they had the week prior. This time, 2489 children responded to the follow-up questionnaire, so around 2/3 of the original group. When they tallied up the numbers, they found that about 13.9% of the adolescents were actively suffering from acne (had at least one new pimple in the previous week). When they further split the groups by dairy intake, they did find that individuals who consumed more dairy products were at a higher risk of developing acne.

The adolescents who drank two or more glasses of full-fat milk daily had a 47% higher risk of developing acne when compared to individuals who did not consume any dairy products. Similar results were found for skim and low-fat dairy products. There was a 29% increase in acne cases in those who regularly consume skim dairy products when compared to those who don't drink any such food items. What's more, the research also found that girls were especially susceptible to the effects of dairy consumption, with a 75% relative risk increase in full-fat dairy consumers and a 47% increase in skimmed dairy products users [112]. In short, the study showed that regularly eating *any* dairy products, including skimmed milk, significantly increases the chances of developing acne.

Another two-part study found similar results, this time performed by a group of Harvard researchers, which used data from the *Growing Up Today Study* (GUTS). If you live in the United States, you've likely heard about this program or even participate in it. The acronym might be unfortunate, but the data gathered through this study is invaluable. This program aims to follow people from a young age into adulthood to monitor their health, dietary preferences, and differences in environmental factors. This way, we can gain insight into whether lifestyle choices made early in childhood can have repercussions later in life.

The study collects data from around 26,000 participants each year, making it one of the largest of its kind. The first iteration happened in 1996, meaning that the earliest participants are now well into adulthood, and some even have families of their own.

The Harvard researchers used this study group to try and find associations between dairy consumption and acne predominance. First, they started with the female participants, examining a total of 3,841 responses. After they analyzed the numbers, the researchers found a link between the quantity of consumed milk and acne incidence. The lowest prevalence was seen in the group consuming less than one serving of milk per week, while the highest acne occurrence was found in the girls consuming more than 2 cups of milk per day. The incidence rate increased linearly with the number of consumed dairy products: the more milk the girls drank, the higher the risk of developing acne [113].

A couple of years later, the researchers moved onto analyzing the records of teenage boys. Once again, the data showed that the lowest prevalence of acne was found among the group drinking fewer than one serving of milk per week, while the highest occurrence was found in the group drinking one serving per day [113]. Interestingly, acne incidence dropped for boys consuming two or more cups of milk per day, but this was still higher than the group that didn't eat any dairy products.

Overall, the data gathered through GUTS showed a significant association between milk and acne, whereby the teenagers who consumed the most milk also had worse acne.

To take it a step further, we can look at studies of studies in this field to see if the results from all scientific papers published so far on this topic agree with each other. This is exactly what one group of researchers did, who looked at and consolidated 14 different research papers that linked acne with dietary factors. This analysis included 78,000 participants, of which 23,000 had acne, while 55,000 were used as control.

Once again, a positive association between dairy and acne was found, whereby people who consumed more milk had a higher risk of developing acne. Patients who were infrequent drinkers of milk (less than one cup per week) had a 24% increased risk of developing acne, while frequent dairy consumers (more than 2 cups per day) has a 43% increased risk of developing acne [114].

Are all these studies conclusive then? Should we consume less than one cup of milk per week to minimize the risk of pimples forming?

Not necessarily. Most of these studies are as accurate as the participants' ability to remember their dietary preferences correctly and objectively assess their acne severity. More so, we can't draw a cause-and-effect conclusion just from epidemiological studies. It could be just as likely that regular milk consumers are part of a higher economic class that can afford other acne-inducing foods, like meat or sweets. To definitively conclude that milk causes acne, we need interventional studies in which dairy products are the only tested variable.

I'm sad to disappoint, but there are no experiments of this nature at the moment of writing. There are plenty of epidemiological studies that link milk consumption with acne, but there are no interventional studies that test only milk in isolation.

Does that mean we can rule out milk as a possible aggravator of acne until we have more evidence? Not necessarily, as we can still check the ingredients of milk. It's not as good as testing it as a whole, but we can nonetheless get valuable clues.

Milk has many different components that can vary between species and farming practices. Still, only a few ingredients make up the majority of milk, so we can start with those.

Take, for example, whey protein, a favorite among athletes around the world. Milk itself is around 3.3% protein, with the majority of it being whey. It's the liquid that remains after cheese production, so it's only available by drinking whole milk and not by consuming derivatives of dairy products, like cheese. If you search for protein shakes on Amazon, chances are you'll land on a product that contains a lot of whey protein, as it's very cheap and easy to manufacture.

Milk-derived protein concentrates have been found to induce many beneficial health effects related to physical performance, including increased muscle mass [115] [116], lowered blood pressure [117], improved recovery after exercise [118] [119], and it even promotes weight loss [120]. It's no wonder athletes go nuts over this stuff.

The reason why whey protein is thought to produce these positive health effects is that, as its name suggests, it is rich in protein and amino acids, which our muscles demand a lot.

In the previous chapter, we've mentioned that mTOR requires two signals to activate: growth hormones and nutrients availability. Amino acids provide the latter. Leucine, a type of amino acid, is a potent activator of mTOR [121], and whey protein contains a lot of it. For comparison, to get the same amount of leucine as two glasses of milk, you would have to eat 130 apples [122] [123]. This is one of the reasons why athletes choose to consume whey protein while exercising: it fires up the mTOR pathway, increasing protein synthesis, thus promoting energy metabolism in skeletal muscle. However, the same mTOR stimulating effect of leucine that improves our physical performance can also aggravate acne.

This link between leucine and acne has been experimentally tested and is well established. A group of scientists from João Pessoa in eastern Brazil sought to find if people who regularly take whey protein supplements are at a higher risk of developing acne. And where better to find people willing to take protein supplements than at a local gym.

The researchers selected 30 participants who had expressed their intent to consume protein supplements. The participants were then followed for two months to see if this dietary change increased the number of pimples. Of the 30 participants, 19 chose whey protein as their supplement. Despite the lack of a control group, the study did find a direct correlation between protein consumption and acne lesion count. After two months on protein supplements, pimples more than doubled in number, both in men and women (see *Figure 4 - Whey Protein effect on acne lesions*). No difference was found between whey and other protein sources [124].

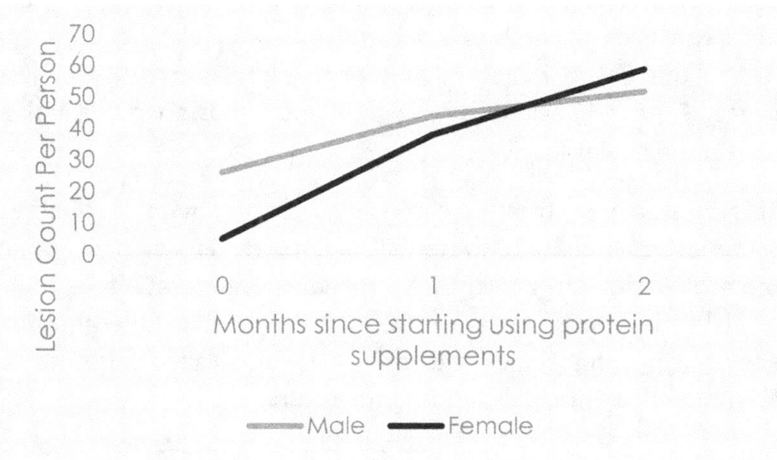

Figure 4 - Whey Protein effect on acne lesions

*

Besides protein, dairy products also contain high quantities of saturated fats, which are also believed to play some role in acne formation. You've likely heard of saturated fats due to their interaction with the good and bad cholesterol and the general health risk they pose. You probably know that unsaturated fats are presumably good for your health, while saturated fats can give rise to certain diseases, particularly heart disease.

The reason why certain fats are good for your health while others should be avoided is due to their physical structure and not their chemical composition, as one might expect.

All fat molecules carry three basic atoms: carbon, oxygen, and hydrogen. They are arranged into a structure that resembles an octopus with only three legs. A fat molecule has a head, called a *glycerol* molecule, onto which three long legs are attached, called *fatty acid chains* (see Figure 5 - Structure of fat molecules). The difference between saturated, unsaturated, and other variants mostly comes down to the fatty acid chain structure.

Some fat molecules have straight chains, while in others, the tails are bent. If all the legs of a fat molecule are straight, then this makes the entire molecule more compact, as it occupies less space. If the fatty acid tails have kinks and bends, then this makes the fat molecules larger.

This difference in structure carries over to the physical properties of foods that contain these fat molecules. Foods high in fat molecules with straight legs (also called saturated fats) tend to be solid, as the molecules are more tightly bound to one another. Foods high in molecules with bent legs (also called unsaturated fats) tend to be liquid at room temperature.

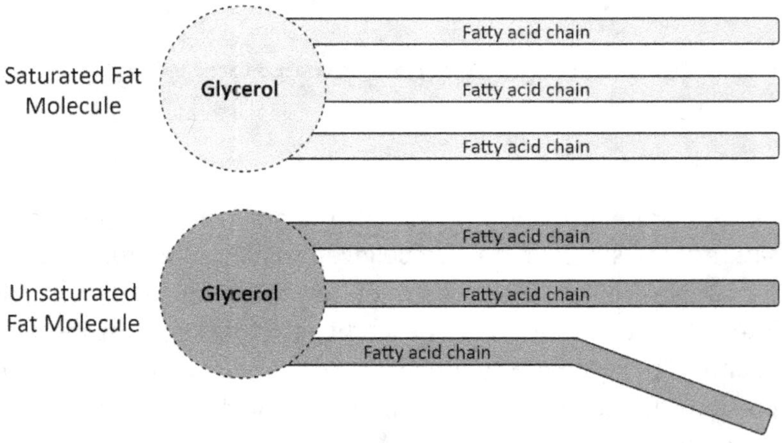

Figure 5 - Structure of fat molecules

The fatty acid chains are comprised of linked carbon molecules to which hydrogen atoms are attached. If all carbon atoms have a hydrogen pair, then this keeps the chain straight. These types of fatty acids are called saturated, as all possible bonds in carbon atoms are taken up (i.e., saturated) by hydrogen atoms. However, if two adjacent carbon atoms have a missing hydrogen slot, this creates a double bond between carbon atoms, causing the entire chain to bend. In this case, the fatty acids are said to be unsaturated, as there are missing slots onto which hydrogen can bond.

Both saturated and unsaturated fats are common in nature. Unsaturated fats are predominantly found in plants (e.g., olive oil), while saturated fats are common in meats and eggs.

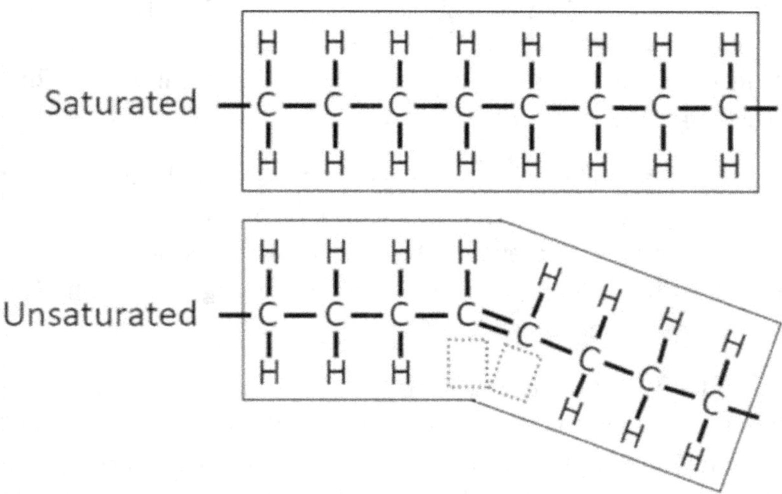

Figure 6 - Structure of saturated and unsaturated fatty acids

The compact nature of saturated fats makes them less permeable than unsaturated ones. This becomes problematic if cell membranes (which are predominantly made of fat) use only saturated molecules. These types of cell membranes block nutrients or signals from easily passing through. A diet consisting only of saturated fats will cause more cells to wrap themselves in these impermeable membranes, making them less healthy overall.

Unsaturated fats are usually cheaper to produce, as they can be harvested directly from plants instead of animals. However, because unsaturated fats are generally liquid at room temperature, they are less suitable for food processing, where solids are preferred.

The food industry has found ways to make unsaturated fats more similar in structure to saturated fats, thus developing cheaper ways of making fat-rich foods. By injecting hydrogen atoms into the fatty chains, they straighten the legs of fat molecules, thus turning them into solids. The chemical composition of these artificial fats differs from the naturally occurring animal fats, but they behave as if they are saturated.

Unlike saturated fats, these processed fats still have hydrogen gaps but at diagonal (transversal) positions. Because the hydrogen gaps are symmetrical, it prevents the fatty acid chains from bending, keeping the entire molecule straight, giving them physical properties similar to saturated fats.

These types of fats, called trans-fats, rarely occur in nature, and the human body has few ways of breaking them down. As a result, trans-fats are hazardous to human health, as they increase the blood circulating levels of bad cholesterol (LDL) while decreasing levels of good cholesterol (HDL). Trans-fats have been linked to disorders of the nervous system, breast and colon cancer, obesity, and shortening of the pregnancy period [125].

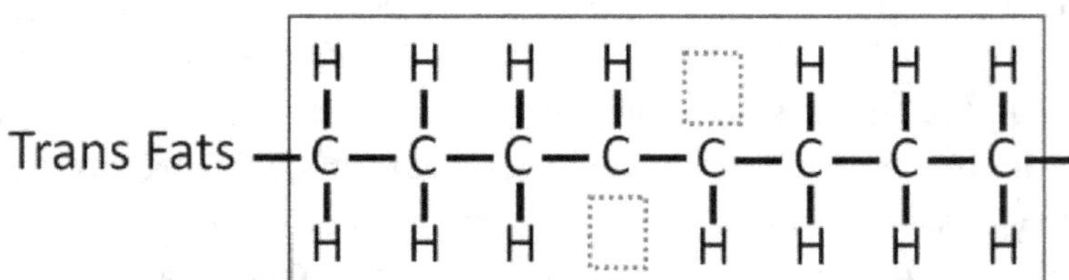

Figure 7 - Structure of trans-fats

Trans and saturated fats also play a role in acne growth. It was found that palmitate – the most common saturated fat – activates mTOR and enhances its translocation [126]. This effect was found to be independent of any other mTOR trigger we've seen so far, including insulin or amino acids. This change in mTOR activity is also quite rapid, occurring within 5 minutes of exposure to saturated fats. Because of this, the saturated fats we find in ultra-processed foods likely play an independent role in acne formation. They can individually activate mTOR through special sensors that look for fat molecules. These sensors are more likely to trigger cell death compared to any other mTOR stimuli, including insulin [126].

Although saturated fats are thought to cause acne, unsaturated fats were found to be protective. They prevent mTOR translocation to the cell membrane, thus decreasing the downstream acne-promoting effects [126]. In other words, the ultra-processed and animal fats commonly consumed in Western diets are likely to cause acne through mTOR activation, while the fats consumed through plants in eastern diets are beneficial to our skin.

Several epidemiological studies have confirmed the link between saturated fats and acne. A survey of Korean dietary preferences found that people with acne consume more foods high in saturated fats compared to those without acne. The foods that were highly correlated with acne are junk food (hamburgers, doughnuts, croissants), processed cheeses, some nuts, and animal meat (pork, chicken) [127].

Another study published in 2014 found similar results. It concluded that people with acne consumed significantly more saturated and trans-fats than average and that acne severity increased the more unhealthy fats were eaten. Patients with moderate to severe acne reported eating twice as much saturated fats and four times as many trans fats as the general population [128]. In both studies, fish was found to be protective against acne, possibly due to its low saturated fat content compared to other food groups. On average, white fish contains only 1.2% saturated fats out of its total weight, compared to 3.8% in chicken, 7.9% in ground pork, 19% in pork belly, and 20% in cream cheese [129].

Milk and especially dairy products are also rich in saturated fats. One stick of butter contains as much saturated fats as 19 cups of sliced avocado, 34 cups of walnuts, or 2,000 apples [130]. The high content of saturated fat in butter is particularly worrying considering that a lot of food recipes start with "melt one stick of butter in the frying pan." Similarly, palmitate (the type of saturated fat that directly activates mTOR) is a major constituent of milk, making up 40% of its fat content [131]. Fat might taste great, but it's not so great for our skin, and especially not for our arteries [132].

*

Although dairy products are rich in mTOR-promoting proteins and fatty acids, we still haven't mentioned the most worrisome of all ingredients. Milk is a cocktail designed to help babies grow, and it's incredibly nutritious at that young age. It contains a wide range of vitamins, amino acids, and essential fats [133]. Intuitively, we should be able to reap its benefits even if we drink it throughout our life, replacing the cocktails of multivitamin pills and tablets we usually take. However, there's one slight hitch. We're consuming milk from the *wrong species*.

A human baby will typically take 180 days to double in weight from birth, while a cow infant will only take 40 days. Seeing as calves grow three times quicker than human babies, we would expect cow milk to be three times as potent in stimulating growth as human milk. And we would be right. Cow milk contains three times as much leucine as human milk (leucine is an amino acid that is a potent activator of mTOR).

The link between time to maturity and leucine content seems to hold across many different species. For example, rats similarly take only four days to double in size from birth, and their milk contains eight times more leucine than human milk [134].

For cows, the potency of their milk translates to other nutrients as well, besides proteins. Notably, milk contains high quantities of hormones designed to promote growth, aptly named *growth hormones*. And one specific hormone in this group thought to promote acne is the *insulin-like growth factor* (IGF-1).

Usually, IGF-1 is produced by the liver when it senses other growth signals present in the human body. Although we will talk more about this mechanism in the

Puberty and Hormones chapter, for now, it's enough to know that IGF-1 and other growth hormones are typically secreted during the early stages of our lives to promote systemic body growth and development. IGF-1 affects nearly every cell in the body, stimulating growth in bone, liver, lung, and muscle cells. Without IGF-1, the human body wouldn't reach full maturity, leading to conditions such as Laron-type dwarfism.

The name of this hormone should give some hints as to how it promotes growth. IGF-1 mimics insulin and binds to the same receptors as insulin does. Thus, it provides growth signals to mTOR, allowing cells to expand and multiply, potentially exacerbating acne [135]. Normally, IGF-1 should be secreted only during puberty, the perfect time in which mTOR should stimulate new cell growth. However, our body can be tricked, especially by the stuff we eat, into producing IGF-1 well into adulthood.

Milk is a potent factor that drives the secretion of IGF-1 [136]. One study found that girls who consume less than 55 ml of milk per day (about a shot glass) had significantly lower IGF-1 levels when compared to girls who consume more than 260 ml of milk per day (about the size of an average mug) [137]. Similarly, a study of 2,109 women found a significant positive correlation between milk consumption and IGF-1 blood levels [138]. In yet another study, Mongolian children that had never been exposed to milk were asked to drink 2 cups of UHT milk daily. After a month of regular milk consumption, the children saw a significant increase in growth hormones and IGF-1 serum levels [139].

It's currently thought that the rich protein content of milk is to blame for the elevated levels of IGF-1. Additionally, milk also contains precursors to growth hormones that might artificially inflate IGF-1 [140]. This extra dose of growth hormones comes as a consequence of how the milk industry operates, which requires cows to be kept continuously pregnant to supply a steady stream of milk.

If you didn't grow up on a farm, you might be surprised to learn that cows, just like humans, produce milk only a short period after giving birth. Cows have no use for milk before a calf is born, and there's no point in providing this growth cocktail if the young have reached maturity. Because of this, cows have to be kept permanently pregnant to continue pumping milk.

The milk production in cows peaks at around 3 to 4 months after calving and dries up entirely after approximately 11 to 12 months. Considering that the cattle gestation period takes about 280 days (slightly over nine months), cows need to give birth right before the well runs dry to maximize milk production. Because of this, farmers usually impregnate cows 2-3 months after giving birth, meaning that cows will be pregnant for 9 out of 12 months of milk production. It is estimated that 75% of commercial milk comes from pregnant cows [141].

During pregnancy, cows experience hormonal changes to support healthy fetal development. Usually, these changes are limited only to sex hormones, while growth hormone levels remain steady [142]. However, the dairy industry noticed that if you administer growth hormones to pregnant cows, this increases the size of the newborn calf and overall milk production [143]. As a result, either a high protein diet or synthetic growth hormones are given to cows before and during insemination to increase meat and milk yield artificially. Particularly, *recombinant bovine growth hormone* is a human-made hormone that is administered to pregnant cows to increase milk yield. It is marketed towards cattle farmers in the USA but is banned in the European Union, Canada, and some other countries [144]. This synthetic hormone stimulates the production of IGF-1, thus increasing milk production [144].

Although IGF-1 in milk survives pasteurization, there is limited evidence to show that growth hormones can be absorbed through the human intestinal tract. For this reason, it's unclear if drinking milk with high concentrations of IGF-1 will be damaging to humans. It's up to you if you want to take the risk, but be aware that some of the studies disproving the impact of hormone-enriched milk are funded by the Dairy Industry itself [145].

Overall, milk is the perfect cocktail to wreak havoc on our skin. It contains a blend of proteins, growth hormones, and saturated fats – all of which have been shown to cause acne independently by interfering with the mTOR and SREBP transcription factors. Still, this is not where the effect of milk ends.

Although milk interferes with the master regulator of growth and sebum production, there is yet another key player in the mechanism of acne that can be affected by what we eat. Researchers first discovered this factor in mutated larvae of fruit flies, which had double the lifespan of normal organisms of that species. The gene that encodes this new transcription factor was even initially named age-1 because the only apparent function at that time was to prolong life. How is it that a gene that can double the lifespan of some organisms can also help us prevent acne?

The answer to this lies partly with what we know to be the true function of this transcription factor. In contrast to mTOR that ensures growth and prosperity in good times, this new factor manages critical body functions in troubling times. Both are needed to ensure we live long and healthy.

Human life is seasonal. This was especially true for our ancestors that had to balance long periods of starvation with long periods of prosperity. In good times, mTOR takes over and prepares us for difficult times ahead, repairing the body and allowing organs to grow to maturity. However, when food is more scarce, the human body needs a way to stop all non-critical processes, including the mTOR-driven growth, to ensure our existing nutrients reserves last to the next meal.

In nature, survival trumps everything else. Similar to how martial law takes over when the fate of a nation is at risk, the master governor of survival must override non-critical body processes to keep the individual healthy. Thus, factors that control survival behave as a rheostat of non-essential functions driven by mTOR and SREBPs, diverting nutrients to where they are needed most.

The acne-factors that we've learned so far have a master switch, which can turn off sebum production, inflammation, and excessive cell death. This switch is typically turned on during periods of starvation, but that doesn't necessarily mean we have to starve ourselves to reap the benefits. These switches can be activated even with moderate levels of nutrients intake.

Survival doesn't kick in only when situations are truly dire, but also in day-to-day living, as part of processes that clean and repair our body. However, as modern life gives us an abundance of nutrients and safe environments, body repair doesn't run as often as it should, leading to more human-made diseases, including acne.

The master regulator of survival

Almost 40 years ago, Michael R. Klauss, then working at the University of Houston, Texas, made an interesting observation on a culture of earthworms. The species of worms that were tested measure only 1mm in length and live in most temperate soils, and, due to their small size, they are pretty easy to miss unless you have a microscope. However, they are the perfect subject for laboratory testing, as they have a quick generation time of only 3 to 4 days and are self-reproductive. A single worm can lay 300 to 1000 eggs, making it the ideal species for growing large numbers of test subjects.

In 1982, Klauss observed that eight earthworms from a single culture had unusually long lifespans. When looking at the cause for this longevity, Klauss found that two worms were born from hibernating larvas known to promote longevity. At the same time, 6 developed various mutations that caused reduced food ingestion and digestion [146]. The link between longevity and nutritional intake became apparent to Klauss at that time, as almost all mutations that caused longer lifespans were tied to food consumption in some way. Back then, we didn't have the technology to pinpoint the exact gene which caused this behavior. Still, a rough calculation using the number of mutated and normal offspring in that generation showed that there was a single gene that caused lower food intake and prolonged life.

Six years later, another research center isolated the gene responsible for these effects, giving it the name *age-1* [147]. The researchers observed that a mutation in this gene increased the average lifespan of worms by 60%. Some lived even three times as much as the average worm.

Since this initial discovery, several other genes were found to promote longevity in this worm species. However, the real breakthrough came when researchers found that the lifespan-promoting genes were actually beacons to a single regulator of longevity, later named *forkhead transcription factor* (FoxO). This discovery propelled our understanding of aging, as just a single transcription factor can now explain many changes that occur in our body due to age. In turn, this discovery also gave us hope that by manipulating just a single gene, we could potentially turn off aging, allowing us to live much longer than we do today.

Alas, FoxO didn't turn out to be the fountain of youth everyone was hoping for. Even so, this novel transcription factor still provided to be an invaluable clue as to why we get certain metabolic-related diseases, including acne.

It might not seem like we have that much in common with earthworms, making these genetic discoveries less relevant to humans. They have simpler respiratory, circulatory, digestive, and neurological systems, and they don't get acne. However, we share surprisingly much with more primitive life forms. We share as much as 70% of genetic information with some species of worms [148]. Even if these genes are not identical in humans, they do have analogs that act in a similar way.

The FoxOs transcription factors get their quirky name as they were initially identified in fruit flies, in which a mutation of this gene caused abnormal head development in the form of a fork. Besides this weird mutation, FoxO factors also promote an increased lifespan, similar to what researchers initially observed with the age-1 gene.

Fruit flies in which FoxO factors were artificially stimulated lived 56% longer than their siblings [149]. Similar results were seen in more complex organisms, including mice [150], and potentially humans [151]. Everywhere FoxOs were tested, the same longevity-promoting effects were found.

These genes are present in humans as well. They were inherited from more primitive life forms and have forked into several variants of our own. Humans now have hundreds of genes in the FoxO family, each controlling unique cellular processes, such as cell stress regulation, metabolism, and cell death [151].

Part of the reason why FoxOs promote a longer lifespan is that they are closely intertwined with mTOR transcription factors. We now know that FoxOs regulate mTOR's nutrient sensor, effectively cutting the antennas that sense amino acids. The nutrients signal goes through a long chain of protein interactions before it reaches mTOR. FoxOs intervene in this cascade of protein interactions, preventing some links from connecting [152]. This FoxO-mTOR axis was shown to reduce several age-related diseases in fruit flies and mammals, explaining the longevity-promoting effects of FoxOs [153].

FoxOs act as rheostats that coordinate intracellular supply and demand. In short periods of cell stress, the effects of FoxOs are only temporary and relatively harmless. However, if the stress lasts for a long time, FoxOs move to interfere with the mTOR transcription factors to further control nutrient production and consumption. Because mTOR governs protein and lipid synthesis, FoxOs use this pathway to ensure sufficient nutrients are present in difficult times, to prevent cell damage or even death [154]. It's unknown just how much of the longevity-promoting effects of FoxOs are due to their interaction with mTOR factors, but they are still closely intertwined. One governs cell function in times of prosperity, while the other acts as a gatekeeper in case of stress.

In light of recent studies, it's now believed that FoxOs are key in managing acne as well. Through their interaction with mTOR, FoxOs can dial down lipid production and cellular death. These beneficial effects can happen if FoxOs are allowed to stay inside a cell's nucleus, where the DNA is located and where the gene transcription process happens. If for some reason, FoxOs are forced outside the nucleus, they are rendered inert, unable to interfere with mTOR and other acne-related transcription factors.

It was found that FoxO1 (a specified protein in the FoxO group implicated with mTOR activation) is forced outside the nucleus more often in the cells of acne patients compared to the cells of non-acne patients. When this happens, FoxO1 can no longer interfere with mTOR's nutrient sensor, thus potentially promoting acne [155]. Experiments have measured this effect and found that mTOR is significantly more active if FoxO1 is moved outside the nucleus [155].

Besides the interaction with mTOR, FoxOs also govern other factors that can lead to acne. More importantly, FoxO1 was found to bind to specific genes in the SREBP family that control lipid production. In-vitro tests have shown that, through an entire chain of gene deactivation, FoxO1 suppresses SREBP-1c factors, which are involved in fatty acid production in various tissues, including the skin [156] [157]. This makes sense considering that FoxOs should balance nutrient production and storage. In tough times, cells divert raw material to critical cellular processes to ensure cell endurance. Sebum does not matter that much to the chances of survival of an individual, meaning it can be sacrificed when nutrients are scarce.

If all of this wasn't enough, FoxO1 is now thought to control the production of anti-microbial peptides on the skin [158]. Peptides are a molecule class similar to proteins, which are used to transmit signals between cells and help kill some foreign pathogens, including bacteria and fungi. Because acne forms when bacteria penetrate the outer skin layer, by producing more anti-microbial peptides, FoxO1 can also dull the inflammation response when a pimple does form.

One related study found that FoxO1 activates these antimicrobial peptides in fruit flies [158]. It's unclear if these effects apply to humans as well, but seeing as both FoxO factors and the immune system are passed down to us from simpler organisms, it's entirely plausible that the same link between FoxOs and these antimicrobial peptides also exists in humans.

Although the link between FoxO, mTOR, and SREBPs is complicated, one thing is clear: all of these factors have one common source of activation, namely our diet. As with other acne-inducing transcription factors, FoxOs are susceptible to the stuff we eat. Although many types of nutrients can activate the master of survival, IGF-1 is an especially powerful signal that can over-stimulate this transcription factor.

In-vitro tests have shown that cells exposed to IGF-1 will force FoxO factors out of the nucleus, thus rendering them inert in their ability to influence other acne-inducing transcription factors, including mTOR [159]. This leaves the cell vulnerable to signals that can cause acne, including those that target mTOR and SREBPs. Without the gate-keeping ability of FoxOs, acne can form freely.

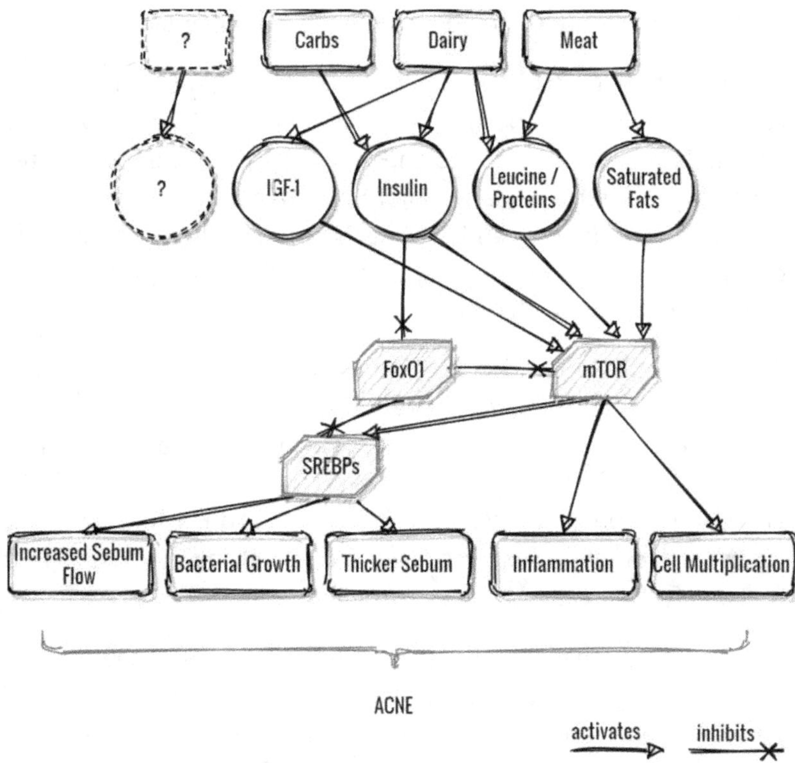

Figure 8 - Effects of milk on mTOR and FoxO1

These observations make foods that increase IGF-1 levels especially dangerous to our skin, and milk is the perfect concoction to cause harm. On the one hand, milk is rich in amino acids that stimulate the liver to produce growth hormones that force FoxOs out of the nucleus [160]. Similarly, milk's high leucine content stimulates mTOR by turning on the nutrient sensor, promoting cell death, inflammation, and lipid production. Lastly, dairy products are also rich in saturated fats, which drive mTOR activation even higher.

As you can see, milk is a potent catalyst that dials up many internal cellular processes that increase our chances of breaking out. It touches nearly every major risk factor for acne, including sebum production, bacterial growth, inflammation, and excessive skin cell death. In theory, milk should be a pimple-pumping machine.

Unfortunately, to date, we don't have interventional studies that can definitely link dairy with acne, but all the evidence accumulated so far points to the conclusion that milk promotes acne. We've seen that many major milk ingredients, from proteins to growth hormones, can harm our skin through several cellular changes. There's no reason to believe that milk as a whole can't have the same impact as well.

The adverse health effects of milk should come as no surprise, considering that it's sourced from species that have evolved to grow three times more quickly and eight times larger than us humans. Moreover, they are excessively fed proteins and synthetic growth hormones to increase milk production artificially. Milk naturally promotes acne, but we are also putting more stuff in it that can further exacerbate the problem.

Are there any other food items that fall in the same boat as milk? For example, soy contains four times as much leucine as milk [161] [162]. Other plant-based protein sources are equally high in leucine, which might also cause pimples to form.

Although there is no direct evidence suggesting soy-based products cause acne, it is known that not all protein sources are metabolized equally by the human body. Protein derived from plant-based sources has been found to not be as easily digestible as that derived from animal-based sources, like milk, eggs, or meat.

One study performed on mice found that protein derived from eggs and milk was more likely to increase blood concentrations of leucine when compared to protein derived from plants. The mice that ate plant-based protein sources (like wheat or soy) did not see an increase in blood leucine levels, even though the absolute quantities of ingested leucine were the same between the two groups [163]. This experiment indicates that our bodies might have an easier time digesting protein from animal sources. At the same time, soy-based milk does not raise blood leucine levels, making it safe for consumption when relating to acne.

CHAPTER SUMMARY

- Milk is a cocktail of proteins, growth hormones, and sex hormones, which has evolved to provide the right blend of growth juice to young offspring. However, cows grow three times quicker than humans, making their milk more potent than what we usually drink in infancy.

- The protein in milk contains special amino acids that can easily activate mTOR, promoting inflammation, sebum production, and excessive skin cell death.

- Humans have a set of transcription factors that regulate cell survival, named FoxOs. Their job is to manage stress resistance, cell-cycle progression, and nutrient availability, but they also mediate mTOR and SREBP activation. If FoxOs are allowed to function correctly, they prevent the acne-inducing changes brought by mTOR and SREBP.

- Milk increases blood levels of insulin and insulin-like hormones, which deactivate FoxOs and activate mTOR. These changes amplify mTOR-driven acne factors even more.

- Several epidemiological studies have linked milk consumption with acne, while the constituents of milk (proteins, growth hormones) were also found to aggravate acne in isolation.

CHOCOLATE AND COCOA

Chocolate is a desert almost universally loved and which is sold in nearly all supermarkets around the Earth. Some studies have found chocolate to be the most addictive food item you can buy [164], hence why we consume 3 million tons of cocoa beans each year [165]. Yet, although this desert is now widespread in Western cultures, its history is actually quite recent.

Ancient Mayans were cucú for coco, consuming it as a hot beverage mixed with cinnamon and pepper, around 400 AD [166]. It was so popular that it was often called the "Food of the Gods," favored by peasants and emperors alike. Aztecs also held cocoa beans in high regard, so much so that they even used them as currency [167]. The plant, as we know it today, doesn't exist naturally in the wild, but it is the result of artificial selection that started some 35,000 years ago in the Americas.

Because this plant doesn't grow naturally in the wild, it had to be imported into Europe after Columbus's famous discovery in 1492. Ten years after Europeans set foot in the Americas, the first encounter between Western civilization and cocoa was made on the island of Guanaja, Honduras. For some years after the initial discovery, Europeans continued to consume cocoa as a beverage, with added spices and sugars. It wasn't until the late 19th century that the solid cocoa bar was invented, giving rise to the chocolate industry as we know it today [167]. Now, we have many varieties of chocolate bars that satisfy even the most diverse taste buds. Some bars are high in cocoa, giving them that distinct, slightly bitter taste, while other chocolate candies contain no cocoa whatsoever.

Not only is chocolate very addictive, but it has also gained a bad rep recently, being portrayed in the media as something that can cause obesity and high blood pressure due to its high sugar and fat content. The research in this area is also quite gray. Some analyses have shown chocolate to be beneficial to our health [168], while others have shown the complete opposite effects in certain dosages [169]. Some people also swear that they break out after eating a bar of chocolate, leading some acne sufferers to give up this sweet completely [170].

Even before reading through the first few chapters of this book, there's a high chance that you already knew that acne is in some way influenced by what we eat. If you have acne, you've probably already tried to alter your diet in some way. Eating less dairy, avoiding fast food, or even drinking fewer fizzy drinks – they all are common dietary changes acne patients try in hopes of improving their condition. As it turns out, the belief that acne is tied to diet in some way is quite common.

In one study, 50 acne patients were asked to describe their personal views relating to diet and acne. In this survey, 92% of responders supported the claim the acne is in some way aggravated by what we eat, with some food items being singled out for having a particularly potent effect. Chocolate came at number one in the list, where 53% of respondents believed that it could worsen acne. Other items high on the list were dairy products (47% of responders agreed that dairy exacerbates acne) and soda drinks [170]. It's no wonder that the majority of the interviewees had altered their diet in some way to try and alleviate their acne. The study also found that only 49% of the participants performed some kind of personal research before committing to these dietary changes, showing once again that most people prefer to go by gut and personal experiences rather than scientific research.

If you're one of the 49% who has tried to research the topic of acne and diet, you might have found that obtaining any credible information on the internet is quite difficult these days. Research papers tend to get misquoted or misinterpreted a lot, either intentionally or not, giving way to plenty of conflicting, incomplete, or downright false information. To create articles on the internet, you don't have to write correct or insightful information; all you need to do is appeal to the masses and be placed high up in the search rankings. Very few of us follow the cited research paper (if present at all) to see if the claims are factual, and even fewer of us perform any critical analysis over said report to see if it has any flaws in its design.

It's not anyone's fault; time is limited, and not everyone can afford to spend hours reading through research papers and decipher their incredibly incomprehensible vocabulary. At some point, you have to trust someone. All of this means that, even if you do personal research on some topic regarding acne, chances are the information you will find will not be entirely factual.

The notion that diet has some effect on acne (be it beneficial or not) dates back quite a few decades. Some initial research on chocolate was done as early as the 70s. One such study, published in 1969 and which is still quoted today, claims that chocolate on its own does not increase the likelihood of developing acne [171]. The 65 subjects who participated in this experiment were fed either regular chocolate bars or bars that looked like chocolate but which did not contain any cocoa. Both candy bars amounted to approximately 1,200 calories per day. This study ran for just one month, during which the severity of acne was observed weekly in all patients.

After the trial period, no difference was found between the two groups. Neither the patients who took regular chocolate or those who were fed fake chocolate bars saw any improvement or regression in pimple counts [171].

This conclusion was pretty definitive at the time and has since become a core research paper quoted in blogs and news reports alike. If you read an article on the internet discussing the effects of chocolate on our skin, chances are the original cited source is this very same research paper.

If you use a popular search engine to read about this subject, at first glance, it might seem that chocolate is harmless, as 8 out of the first 10 search results conclude that chocolate does not affect our skin. However, if you follow the original quoted research paper for each search result, 7 of them point to the study performed in 1969. Even though more internet articles claim that chocolate is safe to eat, they all base their conclusion on just a single experiment completed 50 years ago.

If this research paper is so often quoted even today, then its conclusions must be correct, right? Seeing as so much time has passed since the original study was performed, if it had any flaws, they should have been uncovered by now, and news sites should have stopped quoting it. Sadly, there is one subtle flaw with this study, making its conclusions questionable at best.

In modern medical research, when testing the effectiveness of a drug or treatment, one must take special care to compare the remedy to a well-designed baseline. Otherwise, you won't know if any change in health is due to the tested drug or because people naturally tend to get better on their own (or simply by chance).

To give an example of why not having a baseline can lead to wrong conclusions, you might have heard from your grandmother that garlic is a sure way to fight common colds. To put these claims to the test, you might go to your local hospital, find ten patients who have recently started showing cold symptoms, and you ask them to take one clove of garlic each day for an entire week. You come back a few days later, and you notice that the symptoms of all patients have improved. You naturally conclude that the garlic cured the patients and that your grandmother is a genius!

At first glance, your experiment may seem pretty sound. You treated patients with garlic cloves, and they got better. Even if you repeat the experiment multiple times, you will find the same results over and over again, making you more sure that these findings were not due to random chance. However, keen-eyed readers might see this is not entirely true for one simple reason: people with the common cold tend to get better on their own. You could have given patients any harmless food or drink, and they would have been better in a couple of days on average.

The body is capable of healing itself. We have natural defenses against bacteria and viruses. Some treatments might make it seem like they are making us better, when, in reality, it was our body healing itself all along. Still, there is one other weird medical effect, which makes testing medications that much more challenging.

People tend to respond to a drug by simply knowing they are taking it, even if the drug is as harmless as plain water. By the simple fact of telling people you are treating their condition, you can improve their health. Even though this effect is not well understood, it now goes by the name of the *placebo* effect. Any new medical experiment must account for this effect to make sure the treatment is making patients better and not their natural defense systems.

If you're testing a new medication, you must have a separate group of patients who receive an inert substance instead of the tested drug to account for the placebo effect or for scenarios in which people get better on their own. Neither group can know if they are taking the actual treatment or the placebo, not to skew the results.

The study that tested chocolate's effect on acne also had a control group, but one which was cleverly designed to sway the results in favor of the sponsors of this experiment. By reading the fine prints of the research paper, you will see that it was funded by the *"Chocolate Manufacturers Associations of the USA."* Similar to what is happening with dairy products, the chocolate-industry sponsored an experiment to disprove the claim that chocolate harms our skin.

If you were a researcher with questionable morals, what tactics could you use to make chocolate look better than it actually is? One simple solution is to compare chocolate to something so unhealthy that it's near impossible to get a bad result. If you look at the ingredients of the bar given to the "control" group, you will see that the fake chocolate was so full of saturated and trans-fats that it would have been near impossible not to cause some adverse health effects (see

Table 1- Chocolate bar study - composition).

The control chocolate bar was made of 28% trans-fats, while the normal chocolate bar had absolutely no trans-fats. We've already established that trans and saturated fats aggravate acne by stimulating mTOR and microbial growth. This makes it very plausible that the unhealthy ingredients found in both candy bars overshadowed the unique elements of regular chocolate.

Composition (%)	Control (fake chocolate)	Treatment (typical 10% chocolate bar)
Chocolate liqueur	0.0	11.0
Cane sugar	53.0	50.0
Nonfat milk solids	14.0	12.7
Milk fat	0.0	5.3
Cocoa butter	0.0	20.0
Trans-fat	**28.0**	0.0
Other ingredients	5.0	1.0

Table 1- Chocolate bar study - composition

The experiment's intent was likely to compare chocolate bars to candy that is similar in composition but lacks cocoa. Although this could have been valid research on its own, a more relevant approach would have been to compare chocolate bars to an average diet. In this case, a control bar would have contained all the nutrients from a typical healthy diet: proteins, fibers, carbohydrates, and a complete vitamin set.

Even so, the original researchers chose to test a chocolate bar that contained very little cocoa. Only 10% of the chocolate bar's weight was cocoa, which makes it more similar to white chocolate instead of milk or dark chocolate. All of this means is that the researchers didn't test the effects of chocolate on acne. Instead, they compared one high-fat candy bar to another high-fat candy bar. It's no wonder that the results were neutral.

Despite its flaws, this paper convinced so many people that chocolate is harmless that scientists simply stopped investigating this topic any further. If you search through www.ncbi.nlm.nih.gov (a database of medical research) for studies on acne and chocolate, you'll only find about four papers at the time of writing. If the intent of this experiment was to confuse and prevent further research on this subject, it certainly seems like it has succeeded.

If we want to find the truth about chocolate and cocoa, we need to look at other, better-designed experiments. In a more recent study, 3775 adolescents from Norway, aged 18 to 19, were asked to fill out a form informing researchers of their acne severity, alongside any diet or environmental factors that might be associated with their illness. Around 12% to 14% of the adolescents were suffering from acne when the study was performed.

After analyzing the responses, the researchers found a positive correlation between chocolate consumption and acne [172]. Interestingly, the study also showed that a high intake of potato chips and low consumption of raw vegetables were positively associated with acne. We've already learned about the effects of fast carbs on mTOR and acne, so these results align with our expectations.

A similar study, this time performed in Turkey, investigated the dietary and lifestyle preferences of 3826 acne patients and 759 clear-skin individuals. The aim was to find any factors that were associated with an increased risk of developing acne. This study also had similar results, in that acne sufferers were more likely to consume chocolate [40]. As in the previous survey, this one found other factors, besides chocolate, that might aggravate acne, including being more stressed, drinking more processed juice, and having a family history of acne. Interestingly, this survey found that some food items might be protective against acne, namely white rice, watermelon, and whole-grain bread.

Although these two studies agree with each other, we shouldn't throw chocolate out the window just yet. As with the other food groups mentioned in this book, if acne and chocolate are associated, that does not mean one causes the other. It's just as likely that people who can afford to regularly consume chocolate can also afford other acne-inducing foods, like protein-rich meat, sweets, and dairy products. There can be a third invisible factor, which causes both acne and high chocolate consumption. To know for sure if chocolate causes pimples, we would need to test the ingredients of this sweet in isolation.

If we were to design such an experiment, which ingredients of chocolate should we test first? After all, chocolate bars do not have a standard recipe; you can make thousands of variations using just four basic ingredients: cocoa, sugar, butter, and spices. We already know sugars and dairy products cause acne, so, for simplicity, we can look at the ingredient that is unique to this desert, namely cocoa.

One potential issue with testing cocoa on its own is that it's quite easily distinguishable from other food items. This makes the placebo effect especially strong, as people already have some notion that chocolate is linked with acne.

To get around this issue, a group of researchers took pure cocoa and filled opaque pills with it. This way, the patients had no way of guessing which treatment they were getting (unless, of course, they split open the capsules before taking them). One group of patients received the cocoa-filled pills, while another group, acting as the control, received a type of gelatin powder thought to be neutral regarding acne. A third group received a combination of gelatin powder and cocoa to see if lower concentrations of cocoa can also exacerbate acne. All pills looked the same, with no risk of patients knowing in which group they were assigned to, thus mitigating the placebo effect.

For this study, patients received a one-time dose of these pills at the beginning of the experiment. The group taking the highest dosage of cocoa ate the equivalent of 5 medium-sized chocolate bars or about 170 grams of pure cocoa. After a few days since taking the pills, the researchers measured the number and severity of pimples in each group. Because patients ingested these pills only once at the beginning of the experiment, this study tested situations more similar to one-time binge eating, as opposed to regular chocolate eating.

What the researchers found was that cocoa does indeed exacerbate acne. By day four, after eating the cocoa pills, the patients in this group had over two times more acne lesions when compared to the gelatin group. The same was true on day seven when the experiment ended. All patients saw a slight improvement at the end of the trial compared to day four, indicating that the effects of chocolate are temporary. But the cocoa group still had significantly more pimples, even a week after consuming the cocoa pills.

What's more, the researchers also found a correlation between the quantity of consumed cocoa and the number of lesions. The more cocoa the patients ate, the worse the acne got [173]. However, this doesn't necessarily mean that dark chocolate will give you more pimples compared to milk chocolate. The experiment didn't check other acne-inducing ingredients commonly found in chocolate bars. The ones in milk chocolate (like saturated fats or sugar) might be even worse for your skin.

It should be noted that women were explicitly excluded from the study to account for any hormonal changes during the experiment. The study size was also quite small, with only 13 participants. Furthermore, most people don't consume five chocolate bars all at once. These shortcomings mean that the results are not 100% conclusive and that chocolate might still be safe if you eat it only occasionally and in small quantities.

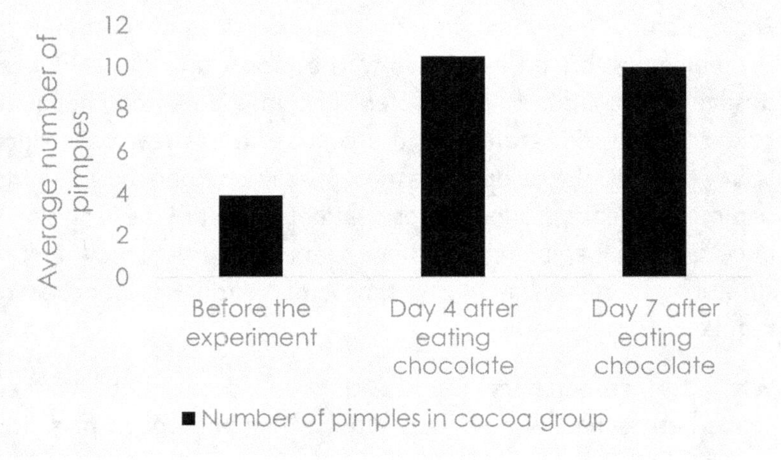

Figure 9 - Chocolate effect on acne

To find out whether temperated chocolate consumption can be equally as bad for our skin, another group of researchers devised an experiment to test regular dark chocolate consumption over four weeks. The researchers chose jellybeans as a control, as they provide the same glycemic load as the chocolate bars, thus neutralizing any potential adverse effects the sugar found in chocolate could have on acne.

Unlike the previous study, this one set out to compare the long-term effects of eating chocolate, as it was performed over a longer timespan, lasting four weeks instead of just one. The patients were also asked to consume significantly less chocolate compared to the previous study, eating only 25g of 99% chocolate daily.

After the trial period, the researchers found similar results to the previous analysis, in that cocoa aggravates acne. Chocolate eaters had twice as many pimples compared to the jellybean group. Interestingly, pimple counts exploded during the first few weeks of the experiment but gradually plateaued towards the end [174]. This might indicate that the human body adapts in some way to the extra cocoa we ingest, adding some tolerability to the extra sweets. It's not known whether we would ever become immune to the effects of cocoa if we consume chocolate long enough, but the current study indicates at least that the adverse effects dull down over time.

As with the previous experiment, only men participated in this study to account for any hormonal fluctuations. This puts into question whether these effects would carry over to women as well. Also, the researchers made no special effort to hide the food items that were tested. If you were a participant, it would have been pretty obvious that you were eating chocolate or jelly beans, making you susceptible to the placebo effect. Either way, seeing as these two experiments agreed with one another, the evidence against cocoa and chocolate is pretty strong.

*

These results are pretty strange when you consider that cocoa is rich in organic molecules found to have a wide range of health benefits. Flavonoids – a set of organic molecules found in veggies, fruits, and tea – are generally considered good for your health [175] [176] [177] [178], and cocoa is rich in several such substances [179]. It's certainly counter-intuitive that something which was found to be anti-oxidative, anti-inflammatory, anti-mutagenic, and anti-carcinogenic can be so bad for our skin [175]. More so, because cocoa is so rich in flavonoids, dark chocolate is now considered a "health food," linked with numerous health benefits [179].

The answer to this enigma likely lies with our immune system. Chocolate can make it hyper-active, worsening the inflammation response once pimples form and bacteria seep deep within our skin.

We've previously seen that certain signaling proteins direct the immune system to the site of injury by opening up blood vessels, thus letting more blood flow to the affected area. For acne, this can happen when the outer skin layer ruptures from built-up pressure inside skin pores. Once a rupture occurs, bacteria are released within our skin, causing the production of pro-inflammatory proteins.

The most common bacteria thought to cause acne is called *Cutibacterium acne* (or C. acnes). It has been re-classified a few times recently, so you might also find it mentioned under the name *Propionibacterium acnes* (P. acnes). These bacteria thrive in closed-up spaces without oxygen, and they also eat sebum. This makes blocked skin pores the perfect breeding ground for C. acnes, as they provide the appropriate environment devoid of oxygen while also supplying the food.

When skin cells detect C. acnes, they release proteins that direct the immune system to where the skin is ruptured. White blood cells start attacking the bacteria, creating the white puss we see when popping pimples.

It's important to note that inflammation happens before the immune system attacks bacteria and before the puss is made. It's very tempting to try and squeeze a new pimple out of existence, but if it's really fresh, the immune system hasn't had a chance to start killing bacteria yet, and all you're doing is pushing the germs even deeper into the skin, potentially making it worse.

Controlling inflammatory signaling proteins is vital in reducing swelling and preventing pimples altogether. What's more, there are many different types of such proteins; some promote inflammation, while others suppress it. To prevent highly inflamed pimples, you would ideally want to dial down the pro-inflammatory proteins while also turning up the anti-inflammatory ones. This is exactly what chocolate mediates.

In one experiment, seven healthy volunteers were asked to consume 50 grams of chocolate containing 30% cocoa. Blood samples were taken from the participants before and after eating chocolate. These samples were then exposed to the C. acnes bacteria 24 hours after they were collected. Through this experiment, the researchers wanted to see if, by eating chocolate, more pro-inflammatory proteins are released in the blood of the participants, thus potentially making pimples worse.

The researchers found that the quantity of pro-inflammatory proteins increased dramatically in the samples taken after the participants ate chocolate. Blood cells containing cocoa flavonoids released twice as many pro-inflammatory proteins when compared to the non-cocoa samples [180]. This effect likely explains why we see an increase in pimple count in people eating chocolate. Your skin becomes more sensitive to the acne-promoting bacteria after you eat chocolate, increasing the odds of local inflammation around skin pores.

Through the previous experiment, the scientists wanted to simulate what would happen in a real human body after eating chocolate. This type of experimentation is called in-vivo (within the living) and is generally more relevant to our health, as it accounts for all the complex systems that make us up. However, it's also harder to pinpoint what causes these changes in our bodies exactly.

In our case, chocolate must first pass through our digestive system, survive the liver, and eventually make it to the skin. These intermediate layers can dilute the effects of chocolate or transform it completely, making it harder to isolate the exact ingredient of this sweet that is to blame for the added pimples. Because of this, scientists usually start with in-vitro experiments (within the glass), where only the active ingredient is tested directly on samples of cells instead of going through the entire digestive tract. This makes the results less relevant to humans but can still provide valuable clues nonetheless.

As part of the same experiment involving chocolate, the researchers also performed more controlled tests on isolated cells. They took a small sample of blood cells and directly applied chocolate flavonoids to them, bypassing the entire digestive system.

After stimulating the blood samples with the C. acnes bacteria, the researchers once again observed the same response as in-vivo tests. Pro-inflammatory proteins were released in higher quantities if the cells were first exposed to chocolate flavonoids [180]. This means that both in-vivo and in-vitro tests agreed with one another. Chocolate tends to cause a worse inflammation response, making our skin more prone to breaking out if we eat sufficient quantities of cocoa.

At this point, the evidence against chocolate is pretty strong. Epidemiological studies have found that people who eat chocolate also tend to get more acne, and we also have a plausible explanation for why this might be. Chocolate is filled with acne-inducing ingredients, such as the mTOR stimulating sugars and fats, and the inflammation-promoting cocoa. If you're not willing to give up on chocolate completely, switching to similar tasting desserts but which have fewer sugars, fats, and cocoas – such as vegan brownies – is likely your best bet.

CHAPTER SUMMARY

- Chocolate has been directly linked to acne through several epidemiological studies, which found that people who eat more cocoa-based products tend to have worse acne.

- Clinical trials have shown that both one-time binge eating and regular chocolate consumption will cause more pimples to form.

- In laboratory tests, cocoa was found to promote the release of pro-inflammatory proteins in blood cells exposed to the acne bacteria. This can increase the odds of pimples forming, as chocolate can make our skin more prone to inflammation once bacteria seep deep within skin pores.

SUNFLOWER SEEDS

For thousands of years, humans have bent nature to provide more food and of higher quality than what we would otherwise find naturally in the wild. Each generation, we've selected the tastiest apples, the largest watermelons, and the prettiest roses to create Frankenstein creations that wouldn't exist without human intervention. This is an excruciatingly slow process that had to be carried through multiple generations until any change was apparent. However, with modern advances in genetics, we can bend nature to our will much quicker, in timeframes as short as years or even months.

Most of what we eat can't survive on its own in the wild, and some species of plants can't even reproduce. Most people wince when they hear the term "genetically modified organism," but nearly everything we eat has been artificially modified in some way. If you go into any of the still surviving virgin forests, you'd be hard-pressed to find wild tomatoes or corn which looks even remotely similar to what we eat today.

Intuitively, it makes sense for us to be wary of artificial plants or animals. Humans have evolved alongside nature in its purest form. For hundreds of thousands of years, we got our nourishment from wild plants, fruits, and certain animals. Our digestive system is fined tuned to extract the maximum nutrients from these food groups and protect ourselves against common toxins. For example, cyanide is a well-known toxin, which can be fatal in humans if ingested in sufficient quantities. It is also used by some plants – including apples – as a defense mechanism against pests. Despite cyanide's toxicity, humans have evolved several ways to deal with the normal cyanide levels we might get from our diet [181], enabling us to eat more sources of foods that would have otherwise been poisonous to us.

If we artificially alter the characteristics of certain plants or animals and then introduce them into our diets, we might create compounds that can't be naturally assimilated by the human body and thus become toxic. Suppose we make apples tastier or larger, but we also accidentally increase the concentration of cyanide beyond the levels that we can safely digest.

These concerns are valid, but we are way past the tipping point. Nearly everything we eat has already been modified genetically in some way, either through selective breeding or through artificial gene splicing. Wild corn, beans, lentils, apples, bananas, and lemons look nothing like their naturally occurring cousins. The same is true for the animals that we eat every day, like pigs, cows, chickens, and ducks. All in all, there are hundreds of domesticated species of plants and animals that humans have altered through selective breeding.

We can also add sunflowers to the list of human-altered organisms. This crop has been modified over thousands of years through selective breeding to yield the maximum oil quantity. We believe that modern sunflowers originated from native American cultures some 6000 years ago, being used in cooking, sunscreen, hair decoration, and medical purposes [182]. Today, it is the fourth most important crop globally, behind palm, soybean, and rapeseed [182].

The popularity of sunflowers can also be explained by their tolerant growing condition, as they are not too picky regarding the climate in which they can grow. Their seeds are also rich in oils, providing a cheap source of fats that can be used in a wide range of food dishes. Approximately half of the weight of a single seed is fat, but that can vary greatly between species. Through modern artificial selection, we now have many variations of sunflowers that were engineer to produce either lots of oils, proteins, or carbs.

The oil we use for cooking comes from pressed sunflower seeds. This, too, can differ in composition depending on the species of plant that is used. This is because the fats from sunflower seeds mostly come in two forms: *linoleic acid*, *oleic acid,* or a combination of the two. Some domesticated species of sunflowers will yield more of the former, while others more of the latter. Standard cooking oil extracted from sunflower seeds is comprised of approximately two parts linoleic acid to one part oleic acid. These two fatty acids are the reason why we suspect sunflower seeds to affect acne, as the oils were found to interact with the human immune system.

Linoleic acid is one of two known fatty acids that are essential to humans, meaning our body cannot naturally produce it. Similar to the nine essential amino acids, we have to get sufficient linoleic acid from our diet to be healthy. Typically, this is pretty easy to do if you follow a varied diet, as linoleic acid is abundant in all kinds of seeds, nuts, and vegetable oils. This is why deficiencies in linoleic acid are pretty rare in modern times [183]. If we couldn't get enough quantities of essential fatty acids through our diet, we wouldn't have lost the ability to synthesis them ourselves.

Although deficiencies of linoleic acid are pretty rare, a high intake of this essential oil has been found to have some positive effects on our body. Particularly, research has shown that foods rich in linoleic acid can have anti-inflammatory effects, marking it as a potential treatment for inflammation-driven diseases [184]. Because of this, the first native Americans that first domesticated sunflowers also used their seeds as a natural remedy for certain inflammatory illnesses [182].

Linoleic acid can also be converted by our bodies to other types of fatty acids. Some of them can have an even more potent effect on our immune system. For example, through a process called *desaturase* (removing hydrogen atoms from a fatty acid), linolenic acid can be converted to *gamma-linolenic acid* (GLA). In turn, this substance has been shown to have an even more potent anti-inflammatory effect compared to the raw building material [185].

Because linoleic acid and its derivatives have been shown to have positive effects on inflammation, we should expect that sunflower seeds can improve acne, considering that pimples are primarily caused by inflammation in the skin. Yet, surprisingly, although laboratory tests on GLA alone were promising, experiments on whole sunflower seeds showed the exact opposite to what we would expect.

In one study, ten acne patients were asked to consume 320 milligrams of GLA daily for 12 weeks while also refraining from using other products that might interfere with acne lesions. After the trial period, the average pimple count went down from 36 to 24 per patient, and sebum secretion was reduced by an average of 15% per patient [186]. This is in line with our expectations regarding linoleic acid and its derivatives. Pure GLA has anti-inflammatory effects, thus reducing the severity of inflamed pimples.

Another similar experiment compared the efficacy of omega-3 fatty acids to that of gamma-linolenic acid as a potential treatment for acne. The hope was that these essential oils could reduce inflammation enough to lessen the risk of pimples forming.

The study itself took 45 participants and split them into three groups. The first group of patients was instructed to consume 2000mg of omega-3 supplements daily, the second group was asked to take 400mg of GLA supplements daily, and the last group was used as the control, which didn't consume any supplements. After the ten-week trial period, both the omega-3 and linolenic acid groups saw significant improvements in acne lesions (see *Figure 10 - Omega 3 and GLA effect on acne*) [187].

In both treatments, the number of inflamed pimples dropped by about one-third, while the control group slightly worsened. After testing the acne patients' skin, the researchers found fewer pro-inflammatory proteins in the group taking GLA supplements, which is in line with our expectations for these fatty acids.

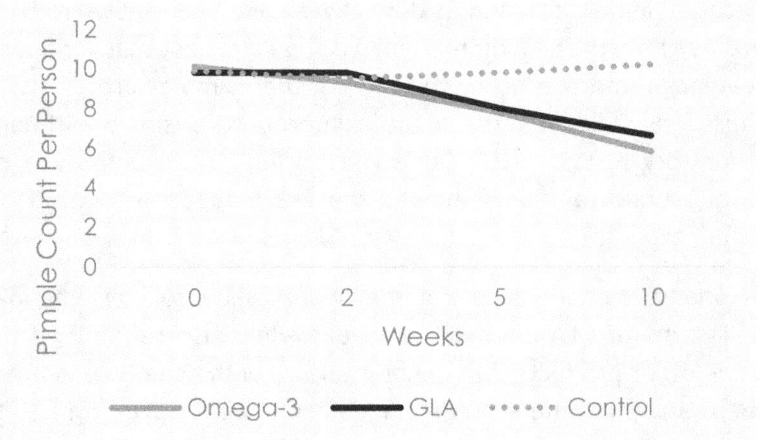

Figure 10 - Omega 3 and GLA effect on acne

Due to the low number of participants in these studies, we can't conclusively say whether GLA can be an effective treatment against acne. However, if you want to try it yourself, blackcurrant seed oil, borage seed oil, and hemp seed oil are all rich sources of GLA. Sunflowers seeds generally don't contain meaningful quantities of GLA, which is why you're better off testing the alternatives.

Because sunflower seeds contain only the precursors to GLA, and because skin cells don't have the enzyme needed to convert linoleic acid into GLA [188], we can likely rule out inflammation as a possible modus operandi for sunflower seeds against acne. There is simply not enough of the good stuff to have a meaningful effect on our skin. But there are other ingredients we can test. Notably, because sunflower seeds are so rich in fats, eating lots of essential fatty acids might change the composition of sebum to make it less or more viscous, thus changing how prone the skin is to pore blockages.

Sebum composition varies by age and gender, but generally, fatty acids make up 10-15% of total sebum by weight. However, it has been found that patients who actively suffer from acne have different sebum compositions when compared to clear-skin people.

In one study, researchers found that the sebum collected from acne patients had 53% fewer fatty acids than average [189]. To compensate and still keep the overall volume the same, the sebum of acne patients had more squalene, which is a substance easily oxidized by the atmosphere and which can cause local inflammation (more on this later in the book).

Many different factors can cause this change in composition. One possible explanation has to do with our diet and the fact that we are not eating sufficient essential fatty acids needed to build optimal sebum. Because we can't naturally produce these oils ourselves, the makeup of our sebum is dependant on our diet. Supplementation with sunflower seeds can prove to be beneficial and restore the ideal sebum mixture.

This is exactly what one group of researchers set out to test. They asked a small number of acne patients to apply a lotion made from linoleic acid on their acne-prone skin. After a month on the linoleic acid treatment, the participants' skin had 25% fewer micro-pore clogs compared to the baseline [190].

The researchers didn't exactly test eating regular food that is rich in essential fatty acids, meaning these positive effects might not apply if we consume whole sunflower seeds. Despite this limitation, the current evidence suggests that acne is partially caused by a suboptimal sebum mixture. Supplementation – especially directly on the skin – can help reduce pore blockages.

What about eating whole sunflower seeds? Do the same beneficial effects apply when seeds have to survive the digestive tract? The amount of linoleic acid that we get from normal quantities of sunflower seeds might not be enough to have a meaningful effect on our sebum, considering that whatever remains after digestion has to be distributed evenly to the 2 square meters of skin [191].

One group of researchers devised an experiment to test the efficacy of whole sunflower seeds as a potential treatment for acne. No more supplements or extracts of sunflowers; this experiment tested the usual seeds that we can find in any grocer. This makes the results more relevant to ordinary people who eat sunflower seeds as an occasional snack.

In this experiment, 50 patients were randomly split into two groups: one consuming normal quantities of sunflower seeds (about 25 grams daily), while the other group was asked to refrain from eating any seeds at all. The study itself took seven days to complete.

After the trial period, the researchers found surprising results that were in contradiction with everything we've learned so far about the constituents of sunflower seeds. Although linoleic acid itself might have beneficial effects, it seems that eating whole sunflower seeds can make acne worse. The group consuming sunflower seeds had more pimples on average than the baseline group [192]. The difference wasn't all that large, only a 10% increase in pimple count. However, that difference grew to about 15% one week after the patients stopped eating sunflower seeds.

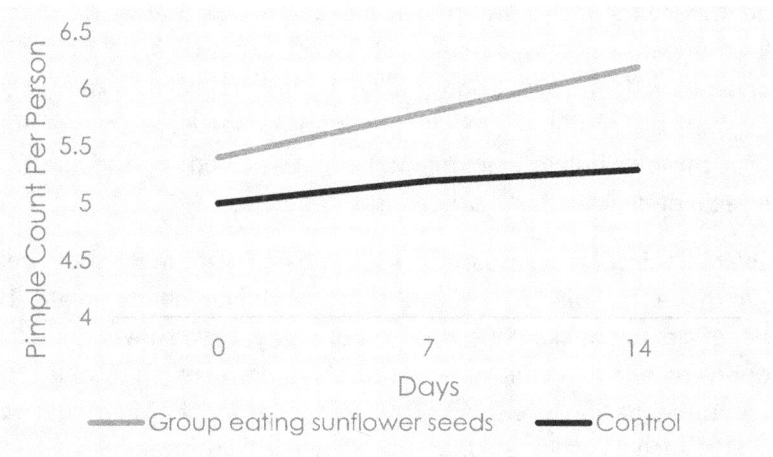

Figure 11 - Effects of sunflower seeds on acne

This shows that in-vitro tests do not always translate to real-world effects when you consider the complexity of the human digestive system and the variety of ingredients in the foods that we eat. Even so, what might explain these strange results?

The short answer is that we simply don't know, and we would need more experiments to help us find the cause. The most plausible explanation for these unexpected results is tied to the other constituents of sunflower seeds besides linoleic acid. Although the original sunflowers were high in linoleic acid, some modern versions of this plant were bred to produce different varieties of oils that are more useful in the food industry.

Notably, the second most common ingredient of sunflower seeds is oleic acid, a type of unsaturated fat, but which has a single kink in the fatty acid group, making it more compact compared to other unsaturated fats.

We know from previous chapters that saturated fats tend to activate mTOR and promote inflammation [55] [193]. Although oleic acid is classified as an unsaturated fat, it's more compact than healthier fats in this group as it has a single kink in its fatty acid legs. Because of this, research has shown that oleic acid can still activate mTOR [194], potentially aggravating acne. This likely explains the conflicting results of sunflower seeds, as any benefits brought by linoleic acid might be outweighed by the harmful effects of oleic acid and other saturated fats.

Overall, the current research puts sunflower seeds in the grey area. We have reasons to believe that sunflower seeds might be beneficial to our skin, but other experiments have shown quite the opposite effect. Until more research is done on this topic, the recommendation is to swap sunflower seeds for healthier nuts and seeds, such as walnuts, which are high in unsaturated fats.

CHAPTER SUMMARY

- Standard versions of sunflower seeds are high in linoleic acid, a type of essential fatty acid that has been shown to have anti-inflammatory properties.

- Derivatives of linoleic acid, such as gamma-linolenic acid, have been shown to prevent inflammation in the skin, thus improving acne.

- Linoleic acid can also change the composition of sebum when applied directly to the skin, further improving acne.

- Despite the promising research done on linoleic acid extracts, experiments done on whole sunflower seeds have shown that acne worsens if we eat the regular seeds.

- The other acne-inducing ingredients of sunflowers can explain these conflicting results, particularly oleic acid, a type of mono-saturated fat.

- Until more research is done on this topic, sunflower seeds should be avoided.

FRUITS AND BERRIES

This book hasn't been kind to foodies so far. As we progressed through the leading causes of acne, we usually came back to the same theme, in that our skin is shaped by what we eat. We've added high-protein, high-fat, and high-carb foods to our do-not-eat list – basically, everything that is tasty. I know that if I were reading this book for the first time, I would be swaying more and more towards medication rather than completely giving up meat, dairy, and sweets.

However, the reality is not that grim. There are food groups that were found to be protective, both to our overall health and against acne. By mixing these healthy foods into our diet, we can likely continue eating the occasional treat, as long as we do so in moderation.

From a young age, you were probably taught by your parents to eat a good portion of veggies with each meal. However, if you were like me, you probably ignored this advice altogether and went straight to the high-fat and salty main dish. Sometimes, we would do everything in our power to skip the main course altogether and go straight for the desert. But, as you aged and become more health-conscious, you likely found that your parents were right. Health specialists and health bloggers alike recommend eating a large portion of veggies with each meal, supporting good health in our years when we don't feel as invincible as we did when we were young. Some people have even switched to eating only vegetables and fruits, thus eliminating some health risks animal products pose.

Our body is fine-tuned to get the majority of nutrients from plant-based sources; it's the way humans have evolved through hundreds of thousands of years of eating mostly foraged vegetables, berries, and fruits. It's the reason we have lost the ability to produce essential nutrients that we would normally get in abundance from our diets, such as certain amino acids, vitamins, or fatty acids. If we break this symbiosis between nature and humans, we give rise to modern human-made diseases. However, if one reverts to a predominantly plant-based diet, it provides the body a chance to reheal and regain its balance. Diets rich in veggies and fruits have been shown to reduce the risk of coronary heart disease [195] [196], kidney disease [197], obesity [198], diabetes, and overall mortality [199].

The same health benefits of following a plant-based diet were found in acne patients as well, and fruits seem to be especially protective. One study performed on 5696 undergraduates found that frequent fruit consumption was correlated with a decreased risk of developing acne. Those who regularly consume fruit had a 14% lower chance of developing pimples [200]. Another study, based in Italy, found that women consuming low quantities of fruit were 133% more likely to develop acne [201].

As we saw throughout this book, if a particular food item is linked with acne, it doesn't necessarily mean that one causes the other. In this case, fruit can prevent acne, but people who eat more fruit also tend to eat less acne-inducing foods, such as dairy, meat, or junk food. To keep a healthy limit on the daily number of calories, you have to eliminate some foods from your diet if you want to incorporate more fruits and veggies. The lack of certain food items may be responsible for the reduced risk of acne, rather than fruits being protective themselves.

The same studies that found that fruit consumption is protective against acne also found that this disease can be passed down from your parents. One study found that you are four times as likely to develop acne if one of your parents had pimples [201]. However, this doesn't necessarily mean that there is an "acne gene." Instead, the reason why acne tends to run in the family may be because bad diets can be passed down from your parents as well. It's nothing irreversible, but a family history of acne or obesity might make it harder to adjust to a healthy diet once outside the parent's nest.

Diets can be inherited from your parents, including bad dietary habits. Although obesity does have some genetic component to it [202], it is still primarily caused by environmental and familial influences [203]. The same is true for acne; parents will tend to pass down their dietary preferences to their children, which might include a fondness for meat, dairy, and sugary foods. The hereditary nature of diets is especially strong between a pregnant mother and her infant.

It was found that many flavors of food can be passed down to the amniotic fluid, influencing neural development during fetal growth [204]. This can program newborns to crave certain foods throughout their life, including those that can cause acne. Once born, the act of breastfeeding is another way parents can influence the diet of their children, as there is evidence that suggests that newborns have some ability to limit caloric intake, but only if breastfed [204]. If milk is provided through a bottle, this reduces the opportunities for newborns to learn how to limit the number of calories they eat, setting up the infant for obesity later in life.

But let's say that, after reading this book, you want to give a plant-based diet a shot. Why would fruits, in particular, be protective against acne? After all, they are high in sugars, which we know to be damaging to our skin.

Although fruits are high in sugar, their influence over acne does not happen through the usual routes we've learned so far, namely the insulin-sensitive mTOR and FoxOs transcription factors. Instead, fruits and veggies help prevent damage to our skin, as they are rich in compounds that neutralize highly reactive molecules created as a result of normal metabolic processes that happen in our cells.

Most people have heard of the term *antioxidants*. We're constantly bombarded with it through all manner of health journals and blogs, which recommend eating more foods high in antioxidants to improve our health. And most of us happily oblige, even if this process is not all that well understood.

Antioxidants, as their name suggests, neutralize molecules that contain unstable oxygen atoms. These molecules are typically created through normal metabolic processes that happen in all living cells, usually through a process called *cellular respiration*. This process converts oxygen and glucose into energy molecules that are used by our cells as fuel. However, about 4% of the oxygen used in cellular respiration is improperly converted into highly reactive molecules instead of energy units, creating waste products that can damage cells in the long term.

These reactive oxygen species (ROS) usually have an extra electron whizzing about in the outer shell, allowing the molecules to interact with most cell components, including our DNA, cell membrane, or other proteins. This reaction is usually destructive and damages the elements that come into contact with ROS. If enough damage accumulates and can't be easily repaired, as a last resort, cells commit suicide to prevent tumor growth and other abnormalities [205]. If enough cells die from this process, it can cause inflammation and general organ failure.

The human body has several mechanisms to deal with reactive oxygen molecules. One of them is antioxidants, which are special compounds that can trap this reactive waste. Usually, our body can produce enough antioxidants to neutralize normal levels of ROS produced through cellular respiration. However, ROS levels can be artificially raised through what we eat or through the way we interact with our environment, overwhelming our natural defenses. If this happens, supplementation with antioxidants might prove to be beneficial to general body health.

Too much oxidative stress can be harmful to our skin as well. The presence of ROS activates a variety of transcription factors that ultimately promote inflammation [206]. We also know that inflammation is one of the first signs that a pimple is about to form, even before bacteria penetrate deep within our skin [207]. If an overabundance of reactive oxygen molecules already stresses the skin, it might increase the chances of inflammation occurring once pimples form.

Another way through which oxidative molecules can cause acne is by altering the sebum composition itself. It was found that squalene – a major constituent of sebum – is oxidized by UV radiation, thus increasing the quantity of ROS in our sebum. The resulting mixture has strong pro-inflammatory properties, irritating the surrounding cells, promoting pimples even without bacteria [208]. This change in sebum composition also makes the overall mixture thicker than usual, thus more prone to blockages [209].

This double effect of ROS has led some scientists to consider antioxidants as a potential treatment for acne. This novel treatment has been put to the test through several studies over the years, and one of the first to do so was started back in 1954.

One researcher took 53 acne patients and asked them to drink two glasses of citrus juice daily. Citrus fruits are rich in Vitamin C, being one of the most potent antioxidants we can eat. The researchers wanted to see if the antioxidants found in standard quantities of citrus juice can have any measurable effect on our skin and if they can prevent acne. After the trial period, 43 patients showed improvements in their acne condition, indicating that antioxidant-rich foods can be beneficial to our skin [210]. Granted, this was a tiny study that lacked any control group, so the results should be taken with a grain of salt.

Although fruits, in general, are high in antioxidants, some, in particular, have shown more promising results in their ability to prevent acne. Antioxidants are one explanation for their apparent protective effect, but the reality is that we simply don't know enough about the complex human digestive and transcription-factor system to understand these effects fully. Either way, let's see some of the beneficial fruits that have undergone the most testing.

Purple Mangosteen

I have personally never heard of this fruit before starting work on this book, and I'm still not entirely sure how I might get hold of it. I'm certain many readers are in the same boat, as this fruit is quite rare in Western markers [211].

The reason for its scarceness is that the mangosteen tree itself is extremely picky when it comes to growing conditions, requiring constant temperatures of above 20 degrees. This makes most of the Earth's arable land unsuitable for growing mangosteen, hence why most of this fruit is cultivated in countries of south-east Asia such as Thailand, Indonesia, Malaysia, and the Philippines. What's more, it can take decades for the first fruit to appear once a new tree is planted. And once the fruits are ripe, they spoil and bruise quite easily, making them a nightmare to transport. Because of these reasons, mangosteen is a very seasonal and expensive fruit, where a kilogram of it can go for upwards of 100$ in Western markets.

Although mangosteen is quite exotic, it has been used as traditional medicine for hundreds of years in the regions where it grows natively. It's been used to treat illnesses such as eczema, skin infection, and even acne [212] [213]. One of the active ingredients of the fruit, α-Mangostin, has also been studied extensively and was found to have anti-skin cancer [214], antioxidant [215], and anti-inflammatory [216] properties. Given these traditional uses and the fact that it's renowned in local culture for its ability to improve skin health, it has also been the center point of numerous studies on acne.

In one such study, a group of scientists took 19 traditional Thai medicinal plans and tested their antimicrobial properties against the acne-promoting bacteria. The researchers found that 13 of the traditional plants decreased the growth rate of bacteria and generally improved acne conditions. The most effective plant on the list was mangosteen fruit extract. The second best was Houttuynia Cordata (more commonly known as "fish mint" or "fish leaf"), but it was less effective compared to mangosteen [217].

Although this study was done in-vitro, the results are promising. Mangosteen seems to have similar antibacterial properties to Benzoyl Peroxide, indicating that it can be used as a topical treatment through creams and ointments applied directly on the skin. This has led some companies to include this fruit as an active ingredient in their products, even if sourcing it is quite expensive. Mangosteen production has seen explosive growth in recent years, with some countries increasing exports 400% year over year [218].

To test the effectiveness of a mangosteen-cream, a group of researchers took ten acne patients and asked them to apply a 1.2% mangosteen gel to one side of the face. The other side of the face was reserved to be the control. Patients were also asked to apply a traditional benzoyl peroxide gel to both sides of the face.

After a 4-week trial period, both sides of the face showed a noticeable improvement in total pimple counts. This is expected, considering that benzoyl peroxide is an established treatment for mild acne. However, the side of the face that received mangosteen extract saw an even bigger improvement, as much as a 50% decrease in inflammation count compared to the region of the face receiving just the benzoyl peroxide cream. Patients also had minimal skin irritation, indicating that extracts of this fruit can be used as valid topical treatments against acne, with fewer side effects compared to conventional drugs [219].

Although mangosteen shows promising results as a safe and natural treatment against acne, this fruit remains quite scarce and expensive. This might change soon as production ramps up in accomodating countries. But, for now, conventional acne treatments remain much more easily accessible and are preferred by most westerners.

You shouldn't be discouraged by this, as mangosteen isn't the only fruit that has shown anti-acne properties. Although mangosteen is one of the best-studied fruit in this group (the majority of research is funded by the Thailand government, which has a vested interest in increasing exports of mangosteen), it's not the most effective or readily available natural treatment.

Barberries

Barberries are yet another less known plant to Western countries, but one which is much more easily sourced than mangosteen and which is significantly cheaper. Barberries thrive in a wide range of climate conditions, meaning they can be grown on all populated continents. Even so, barberries remain an obscure plant to Western markets due to their risk of harboring wheat rust – a fungal disease that attacks mainly cereal plants and which can be devastating to local farmers. Some countries have banned growing this plant altogether, particularly Noth America. But, if you can't grow barberries locally, you can still get bags of dehydrated berries from your local middle-eastern shop or Amazon.

Unlike mangosteen, barberries haven't been used in traditional medicine as much. Some recorded cases in Chinese folklore mention using extracts of barberries as an oral antibacterial, but that is mostly it [220]. Instead, because they have a slightly tangy/acidic flavor, barberries are mainly used for culinary purposes, particularly in middle-eastern dishes.

What makes barberries unique, besides their tangy taste, is their high concentration of the *berberine* compound. It is this very compound that gives barberries their distinctive health benefits. Although barberries are not the only plant that contains this substance, they remain the most accessible source to come by.

Berberine has been studied extensively over the years and is emerging as an exciting compound that promotes a wide range of health benefits. If you search for research papers on this topic, you will find over 5000 different documents that mention this extract.

Berberine's popularity is well deserved. In-vitro tests have shown that berberine reduces insulin resistance, decreases inflammation of vascular cells, is neuroprotective [221], and might even decrease the risk of developing certain cancers [222].

Relevant to this book, berberine has also shown to have general anti-inflammatory and antioxidant properties, thus preventing two of the biggest risk factors for acne [221]. This could potentially reduce pimple severity by dulling down the inflammatory response once pore clogs form. More so, it could also prevent acne altogether by reducing reactive oxygen molecules that irritate skin cells.

Recent studies have also shown that berberine modulates mTOR [223], as well as reducing total sebum production on the skin. Granted, this last effect was observed in mice, but the change in mTOR activation and sebum production was pretty substantial. Mice that were fed barberry extract had a 63% reduction in sebum production on the skin [224].

These potential beneficial properties have also been confirmed through interventional studies. In one such experiment, scientists recruited a small number of adolescents with mild to moderate acne and administered pills containing barberry extract to half of the patients, while the other half received an inert substance. Because the experiment was done in Iran, it was quite easy for the researchers to get hold of these berries by simply going to the local market. They took the store-bought berries, boiled them, and filled opaque pills with the resulting mixture. Both the barberry extract and placebo pills were given to a total of 50 adolescents with acne. They were then followed for four weeks to see if their symptoms improve at all.

As expected, the control group saw no noticeable change in total lesion count after the 4-week trial period. However, patients ingesting the barberry extract saw an almost 50% reduction in pimple count. The decrease also continued well into week four (see *Figure 12 - Barberries effect on acne*) [225].

This study was reasonably well designed, and the results were statistically significant. Although more research is needed to confirm the positive effect, for now, it seems that barberries can be used as a cheap and effective treatment against acne. The dosage of the barberry extract used in the previous study equates to only around 6g (or one tablespoon) of raw fruit per day. Their tangy taste might make barberries hard to incorporate in many dishes, but they go great with breakfast meals, especially oatmeal.

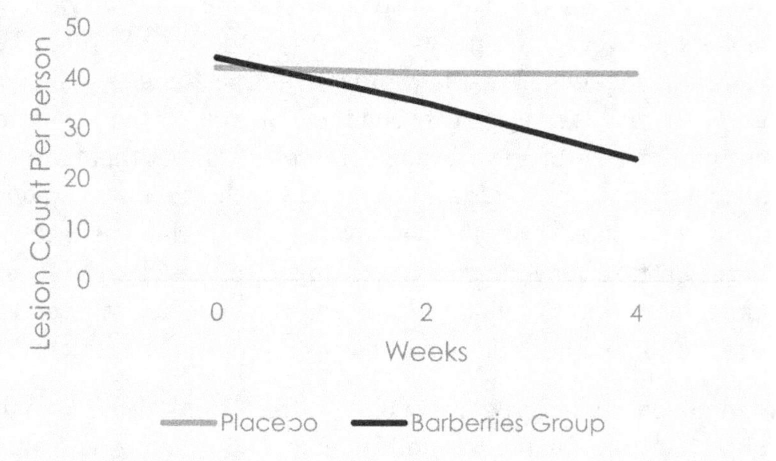

Figure 12 - Barberries effect on acne

Having read this conclusion, you might be wondering why barberries are not recommended more to acne patients and why it remains such an obscure plant. The primary reason is fairly simple: plants can't be patented.

Because you can't put a label on barberries, pharmaceutical companies have minimal incentive to fund research for this plant or promote them as an effective treatment for acne. People can simply run to their nearest store and get bags of this stuff for relatively cheap. This is true for most readily available and inexpensive natural treatments. For example, heart disease remains the largest killer in the US [231], and the most effective way to prevent this illness remains to adopt a healthier diet and increase physical activity [226]. Although a more nutritious diet is thought to be 20 times more protective than even the best commercially available drug [227], a visit to the doctors for symptoms of heart disease will likely result in a prescription for medication instead of exercise.

*

The fruits that we've looked at so far are fairly exotic for Western markets. However, the good news is that the list of protective plants does not end here. Many other beneficial fruits have shown promising results against acne, and there are many others that we haven't gotten around to testing. The reality is that there are so many different kinds of fruits out there – each one with a unique blend of flavonoids, vitamins, antioxidants, and other chemicals – that it will take some time to test them all. This task is made even harder by the lack of funding in this area of human health. Even so, here are some other fruits which have shown positive results:

Mango – an in-vitro experiment using extracts from Mango kernels found that this mixture has antibacterial, antioxidative, and anti-inflammatory properties. This study indicates that mango kernel extract can be used as an effective treatment against acne if applied to the skin [228]. It's unclear if eating mango will have the same positive effects.

Apple – "An apple a day keeps the acne away" is the conclusion reached by one group of researchers after they tested the antimicrobial properties of multiple fruits and plants, including apples [229]. The same study found similar positive effects from **Japanese knotweed, Rhodiola,** and **Hyacinth bean,** indicating that extracts of these plants could be used as topical treatments against acne.

Fig – a gel containing 4% extract of fig fruit was applied on the skin of multiple acne patients to see if it would reduce the rate at which pimples form. Among other effects, this gel was found to significantly reduce sebum production, marking it as a potential topical treatment for acne [230].

Pomegranate – to quote directly from one study: "The antibacterial properties of [pomegranate extract] [...] on the most common bacteria associated with the development and progression of acne suggest that these extracts may offer a better preventative/therapeutic regimen with fewer side effects than those currently available" [231].

Apricot seed – these seeds are frequently used in oriental medicine to treat several skin diseases, including acne. An in-vitro study using extracts of apricot seeds found that this mixture has antimicrobial effects against the acne-promoting bacteria [232].

Fruit Acid Extracts – a group of researchers compared glycolic-acid peels to an extract made from various fruits to see if the two mixtures can reduce the rate at which pimples form. The researchers found that both medicines can prevent non-inflamed lesion count [233]. Fruits that contain large amounts of fruit acid include avocados, kiwifruits, bananas, melons, and strawberries [234]. Chemical peels in general – be it fruit-based or not – should be used only with care. If you leave them on for too long, they can cause severe chemical burns.

The list of beneficial fruits is much longer than this, as many others have shown antimicrobial, antioxidation, or anti-inflammatory properties. Which one is the best is still up for debate, but you can never go wrong with incorporating more fruits and vegetables into your diet. If nothing else, you will have fewer chances of getting heart disease [235], cancer [236] [237], type 2 diabetes [238], and … constipation [239].

CHAPTER SUMMARY

- Cells generate waste as part of the normal cell process that converts glucose into energy. These byproducts contain unstable oxygen molecules and are highly reactive. They can damage cells to the point of causing complete cell death.

- Cells that contain reactive oxygen molecules will release more pro-inflammatory signaling proteins, exacerbating acne. Oxidation can also occur to sebum. If this happens, the entire mixture becomes thicker, thus promoting pore blockages.

- Antioxidants help deactivate cell waste products, acting as "garbage disposal" systems for the cell.

- Fruits and vegetables are rich in antioxidants, and epidemiological studies have shown that diets rich in plant-based foods are protective against acne.

- Some fruits and seed extracts have been shown to have especially potent anti-acne effects. Examples include purple mangosteen and barberries.

HERBS AND SPICES

There's a depressing health trend starting to emerge in recent years, in that some Western countries are seeing a decrease in life expectancy, despite the latest advances in medicine. This can seem quite oxymoronic, considering that these countries tend to have higher health care costs per patient when compared to non-westernized societies.

Take, for example, the United States. It has by far the highest health costs per capita of any other nation on earth [240], but it's ranked only 35th in life expectancy [241]. What's more, since around 2013, life expectancy is actually decreasing year over year [242].

There are many reasons why the US health system is performing so poorly, but the most cited explanations are a growing preference towards fast food (and a generally poor diet), sedentarism, smoking, and psychological distress [243] [244]. Although all of these factors are valid and should be treated with urgency, there's one other aspect that sets the US apart: the cost of the health care system itself. It's quite common to see headlines for absurd hospital bills for the most mundane of injuries, like a 14,000 US dollar bill for a 45-minute hospital visit to fix a cut finger [245], or 2,000 dollars for an ambulance [246]. The issue is so absurd that, in the US, the life expectancy gap between the richest and poorest 1% of the population is estimated to be 14 years for men and 10 years for women [247]. Not everyone is dying sooner, just the poor.

As a result of increasing health care costs, more and more people are either refusing medical treatment until it is too late or are turning towards more alternative forms of care, which are a lot cheaper and easier to come by than regular pharmaceuticals.

Traditional medicine hasn't passed the scientific rigors of modern-day medical testing, but it does have one advantage: thousands of years of trial and error to figure out which remedies genuinely have a positive health benefit. This does not necessarily mean that traditional medicine can't be wrong. It often is more than it's not.

Ancient Egyptians and Greeks used urine to treat acne [248], while Egyptians also believe pimples were caused by lying [249]. We shouldn't use traditional medicine blindly, but it can provide valuable hints as to where to start more rigorous scientific research. We still don't understand a lot about how the human body works, and a good portion of modern medicine was discovered by accident without knowing how and why it works. Viagra, for example, was discovered while investigating ways to treat chest pains. Only after noticing the pleasant side effects in patients who initially tested Viagra did we know about this drug's ability to fuel our love rockets.

The problem with traditional medicine is that we have a vast number of unique concoctions that need to be tested before they can be deemed safe and effective. Considering that pharmaceutical companies have low interest in developing drugs on freely available plants, this makes the entire process extremely slow.

Hope is not lost, as some plant-based treatments are making the transition from traditional medicine to just *medicine.* Sweet worm, for example, has been used as a medicinal plant for thousands of years in Chinese folklore, being used to treat chills and fever. Recently, these health benefits have been confirmed through modern medical research. Nowadays, this plant is sold under the brand name *Artemisinin,* which is prescribed as a treatment for malaria. Similarly, *Khella,* which was originally used as a treatment against asthma in Middle Eastern countries, is now sold as the Cromoglycate drug. Many other medicines follow the same path [250].

This increased interest in traditional treatments is evident not only from the number of published scientific papers that study these remedies but also in the market capitalization of the industry. In 2014, the total herbal medicine market was valued at close to 63 billion USD, while in 2016, it jumped to 71.2 billion USD, a 13% increase in just two years [251].

Some plants and remedies are studied more than others, depending on their availability and how widespread the usage is. Even so, in recent years, one plant, in particular, has spawned an entire cult following, gaining the interest of thousands of scientists. Can you guess what is the most researched traditional medicinal plant?

Green tea takes the top spot, with 34,415 articles that mention this plant at the time of writing [252]. Garlic comes in number two with 6,624 scientific papers [253]. The interest in these two plants alone has exploded in recent years; over 90% of articles that mention green tea were published after 1992. This is good news for us, as green tea has shown remarkable properties that improve our general health and that of our skin.

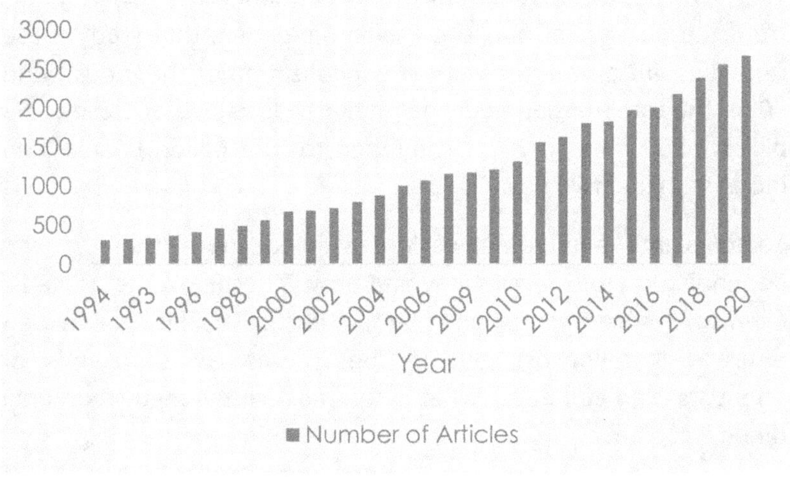

Figure 13 - Number of articles referencing green tea

The recent interest in alternative forms of treatment does not mean we should use plant-based medicine blindly. At the very least, you risk wasting your money on something which has no effect whatsoever. That being said, we should also not discredit treatments that have been proven to work, just because it is not sold in pill form. This includes remedies for acne as well. Some herbs have been used in traditional medicine for thousands of years and, when put under the strictures of modern testing techniques, they hold their value even in modern times. We will look at some of these treatments next.

Green Tea

The human body is quite complex, and we're far from understanding how all the internal pieces work and how they interact with each other. If we did understand everything about our body, we wouldn't need clinical trials to test whether some medicine works or if it has any side effects. We would simply run simulations on a very powerful computer and be done in a few hours. Until we reach that point, any new drug we introduce must pass scientific rigor, especially to test if it has any serious side effects.

After all, you can kill cancer cells in a petri dish using sulfuric acid, but you wouldn't want to drink it straight up. Because the human body is complex and we still have much to learn about its inner workings, if someone mentions that they have found a miracle drug that cures many illnesses with no side effects, you would be highly skeptical. Yet, despite its unlikelihood, there is one medicine that is shaping up to be just that, one which has shown many health benefits, with little to no side effects. And better yet, it's also dirt cheap.

Green tea is a readily available plant that is so essential to certain nations that it even spawned several wars [254]. The famous American independence war was sparked after tea prices skyrocketed due to increased taxes from the UK. Similarly, Britain also fought two separate wars with China over trade disputes concerning tea [254].

Today, green tea is consumed primarily as a beverage, but for most of its history, it was either eaten directly or incorporated as a spice in dishes [255]. It wasn't until the 8th century that we discovered a new way of consuming green tea, by steaming green tea leaves, thus getting a much more pleasant taste. Since then, tea was propelled to become the most popular prepared beverage in the world, overtaking even coffee, with 266 billion liters consumed each year [256].

Despite it being popularly used as a tasty beverage, green tea also has a reputation for being good for one's health, which dates back thousands of years. A Chinese legend states that ancient emperor Shen Nung (a mythological deity) discovered tea while noticing a pleasant aroma after leaves from a nearby tree fell into a cup of boiling water. He then immediately proclaimed the new drink to be "sent by the gods," cementing the belief that it is a cure for many common diseases.

Although the notion that gods created green tea might seem farfetched, recent research into this plant revealed that at least some of the fame might still be well deserved. For example, regular green tea consumption has been shown to improve cognition [257] [258], reduce the risk of various cancers (including prostate [259] and gastric [260]), reduce stress, improve sleep [261] [262], reduce inflammation [263], promote weight loss [264], and many more. Some of these positive effects apply to our skin as well, making green tea a prime candidate as an alternative acne treatment.

The reason why we believe green tea is so effective at treating this many afflictions has to do with certain chemical compounds that are abundant in plants and very concentrated in tea tree leaves. This class of compounds is named *polyphenols,* which have been proven to have a wide range of health benefits. Some of them carry over to green tea as well [265].

Green tea is one of the richest sources of polyphenols that you can consume, second best only to eating tea tree leaves directly. If chewing green leaves isn't your thing, make sure to at least drink green tea, as the oxidation process used to make other types of tea – such as black tea – destroys some of these beneficial compounds [266].

Polyphenols, as a group, have strong antioxidant properties, hence why they have such a wide range of health benefits. Cell damage caused by excessive oxidation can cause numerous health problems, as it can affect virtually all organs. By neutralizing oxidants using the polyphenols found in green tea, you could potentially improve health systematically throughout your body.

Oxidative damage also increases cell turnover rate, as it activates programmatic cell death, causing more cells to be created. We also know that excessive cell production is a leading cause of cancer, which explains why green tea is now believed to prevent certain forms of this disease as well, including lung, colorectal, skin, prostate, and breast cancers [265]. The notion that gods created green tea is starting to sound more and more plausible now.

There are over 500 known types of polyphenols to study, but thankfully only a small number are found in abundance in tea tree leaves and are relevant to our skin. One such compound is called *epigallocatechin-3-gallate* (EGCG) and makes up approximately 10% of the weight of a single bag of green tea [267]. The concentration of EGCG is highest in green tea compared to any other beverage or food item you can eat. You will get about 10g of EGCG in every 100g of green tea that you consume, but only 0.9g in the same quantity of black tea. Apples, plums, onions, and other non-tea sources will give you a measly 0.1g per 100g of food. Green tea is easily the cheapest and most abundant source of this polyphenol.

We're interested in EGCG in particular and not the other 500 polyphenols because this chemical has been shown to improve acne conditions through numerous in-vitro tests.

On the one hand, EGCG has been found to modulate mTOR activity, potentially reducing the risk of acne by dulling down this transcription factor [268]. Interestingly, this discovery was made while investigating the cancer-preventing abilities of green tea and EGCG. The researchers found that mTOR's growth signal is cut-off when in the presence of EGCG, thus influencing several transcription factors in the mTOR activation chain. Although not explicitly tested, the same chain of transcription factors is also involved in the suppression of FoxO1. This means that EGCG likely has a double effect on acne, both dialing down mTOR while also allowing FoxO1 to exercise its mTOR-suppressing abilities.

Besides the mediating effects over mTOR, EGCG has also been found to control other factors that can promote acne. For example, green tea can directly inhibit the gene transcription factor SREBP-1 [269], which influences the rate at which lipids and sebum are produced.

In vitro tests showed that sebum-producing cells treated with just 4mg of EGCG (or slightly under 1% of a cup of green tea) showed a significant reduction in lipid production. This effect was amplified even more with higher concentrations of EGCG. At 18mg of EGCG (or 4% of a cup of green tea), sebum production was halved compared to the baseline cells.

The researchers observed other potentially beneficial changes to sebum, including a reduction of cholesterol and triglycerides compounds. Cholesterol specifically is a solid at room temperature and has a waxy consistency [270], making it much more viscous than ordinary sebum. By decreasing cholesterol concentration, EGCG would also decrease the overall viscosity of sebum, reducing the likelihood of clogs forming in skin pores.

Besides affecting the three main acne-related transcription factors, EGCG has also been found to mediate the immune system, playing an even deeper role in acne development. In the *Chocolate and cocoa* chapter, we've seen how skin cells emit pro-inflammatory signaling proteins when they detect bacteria. Chocolate amplifies this effect, hence why we believe it aggravates acne. EGCG works in reverse by dulling down the inflammation response.

In-vitro tests have shown that skin cells treated with EGCG emit significantly fewer pro-inflammatory proteins when they come into contact with the acne-causing bacteria. Higher concentrations of EGCG induce even more potent protective effects. Although anti-inflammatory effects were found for as little as 4mg of EGCG, higher quantities of EGCG showed even more pronounced changes in the immune system response. For 18mg of EGCG (equivalent to 4% of a cup of green tea), the activity of certain pro-inflammatory proteins was halved [269].

As if all of this wasn't enough, green tea has also been shown to kill the actual acne-promoting bacteria when applied directly to the skin. The strength of this effect also seems to be directly correlated with the concentration of EGCG, suggesting that the more green tea you consume, the more potent the protective effect will be (see Figure 14 - EGCG effect on C. acnes) [269]. At concentrations much lower than a typical cup of green tea, solutions containing EGCG are extremely effective at killing the acne bacteria. When concentrations are high enough, bacteria die off completely.

It should be noted that this effect was observed if the EGCG solution was applied directly to the bacteria colonies. This means that to get the complete antibacterial properties of green tea, you would need to use lotions on the skin to ensure that it comes into contact with the acne bacteria itself. It might not be as pleasant as drinking green tea, but at least tea extract lotions are fairly cheap and easy to come by.

The antimicrobial properties of green tea come from the abilities of EGCG to destroy the protective membrane of the acne-promoting bacteria. Unlike most viruses, a single bacterium is a self-contained unit, having all the necessary biological machinery to reproduce and generate its own energy. This machinery is protected by an outer membrane of lipids and proteins, similar to how most human cells are structured. EGCG can destroy this protective membrane while also preventing its repair, thus leaving all the delicate internals vulnerable [271].

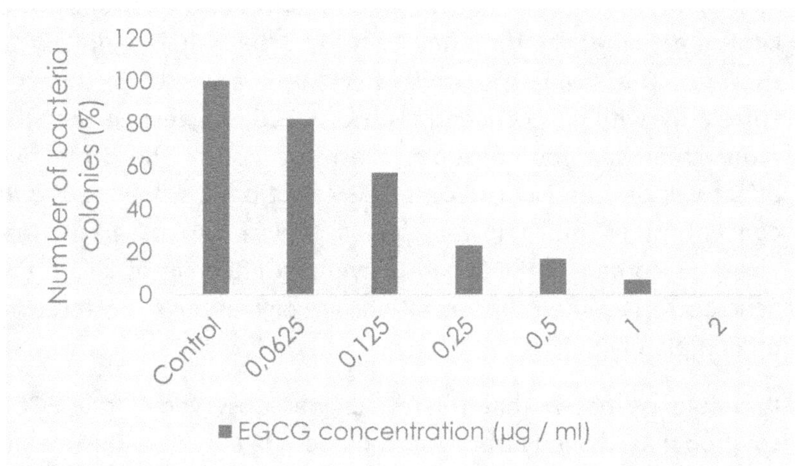

Figure 14 - EGCG effect on C. acnes

At this point, we've seen that green tea improves almost all risk factors associated with acne: it suppresses the cell proliferating effects of mTOR, it decreases sebum production by deactivating SREBP-1, it has anti-inflammatory properties, and it also kills off the acne-promoting bacteria itself. Shen Nung might not have been so far off when he called green tea a godsend.

The caveat to these protective effects is that they have mainly been observed in lab-controlled scenarios. Although the concentrations used in lab tests might seem high enough (1% to 4% of a single cup of regular tea), you should remember that the tea we usually drink has to survive the digestive tract and then be distributed to all cells in the human body (which there are a lot of). After drinking a single cup of green tea, a square centimeter of skin would receive only the one-millionth part of a cup of this beverage. You would have to drink a whole lot of green tea to get the same concentrations in your blood as used in the in-vitro tests.

Despite this discouraging fact, it seems that at least some of the beneficial effects of green tea apply even when drinking regular quantities of this beverage. In one experiment, a group of researchers took regular, air-dried green tea leaves and created a concentrated extract obtained by first boiling the tea leaves (as you would normally do for traditional tea) and then removing most of the moisture from the resulting liquid. This residue was then put into pill form and given to several acne patients to see if their condition improved. The extract taken in pill form was equivalent to approximately one cup of standard green tea consumed daily.

You might be wondering why the scientists went through all that trouble to create concentrated pills of green tea instead of giving bags directly to patients to brew themselves. The answer to this lies with how medical experiments should be designed to account for the placebo effect. Researchers need to take special precautions to hide the tested medicine, not to influence the results of the experiment. If patients know which medication they are taking, they might be especially susceptible to the placebo effect, causing improvements in health even if the pill is inert. Green tea is also quite easy to spot, due to its distinctive aroma, meaning scientists need to take extra precautions to hide it. If you put extracts of green tea into opaque pills, neither the treatment nor the control groups have any way of knowing which drug they are taking.

In the green tea experiment, the acne patients were split into two groups: one taking pills containing the green tea extract and the other taking capsules filled with harmless substances. The acne severity was measured before and after the experiment, which lasted four weeks.

At the end of the trial, the research did, in fact, observe a reduction in acne lesion count in the green tea group by around 27% compared to the non-tea group [272]. The acne patients were not completely cured, but the trend in pimple reduction indicates that the improvement could have been even larger if the trial was any longer. Every little bit helps, and if you can get rid of a quarter of your pimples by simply drinking delicious tea, that's one medicine I would be glad to take.

It should be noted that the current experiment tested unsweetened tea without any added milk or sugar. It's unclear if the same benefits would be seen with tea containing other additives, considering that both sugar and milk were found to cause acne independently.

Drinking regular green tea looks promising, but what about tea lotions applied directly on the skin? We know that EGCG extracts were found to kill the acne-promoting bacteria in in-vitro tests, but would the same effects hold for ordinary people applying commercial lotions of tea extracts?

It seems so. Several trials have confirmed the antibacterial effects of tea tree oil extracts when applied directly to the skin. One study compared the effectiveness of Benzoyl Peroxide – the most common topical treatment for acne – with that of a concentrated lotion made from tea tree extract. Although the Benzoyl Peroxide solution was more effective at reducing the number of pimples, the group applying tea-tree oil saw an improvement as well. The number of acne lesions in the tea-oil group was halved compared to the start of the experiment (see Figure 15 - Benzoyl Peroxide versus tea-tree oil) [273].

Even though the study took three months to complete, the downwards trend continued right until the end of the trial period, indicating that the more you apply tea tree extracts, the better the results.

Other similar studies mirrored these positive effects of tea tree lotion, showing significant improvements in acne patients [274] [275] [276]. However, unlike conventional acne treatments like Benzoyl Peroxide, green tea extracts have little to no side effects. This is a crucial aspect for medications that are used long-term.

If you plan on treating acne using lotions, you must continue using the medication for as long as you are at risk. This can take years of constant treatment. Minimizing side effects for such long-running remedies is extremely important to make sure that the adverse effects do not outweigh the benefits brought by the medicine.

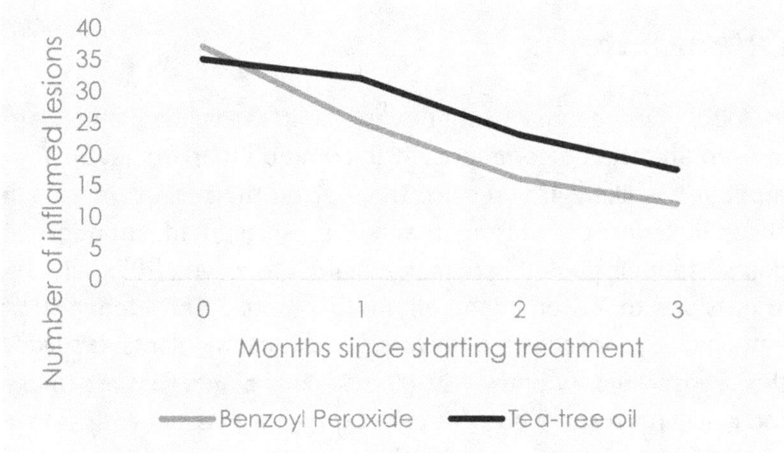

Figure 15 - Benzoyl Peroxide versus tea-tree oil

Considering that green tea is dirt cheap, is already consumed by a large percentage of the population, and has little to no side effects, I recommend giving it a try. To get the full benefits, you can supplement drinking green tea by applying tea tree oil extracts on the face. It's also important to consume only unsweetened tea with no added ingredients to not negate this plant's added benefits.

Besides tea, other plants have shown similar acne-fighting properties, most of them being used as traditional remedies long before modern medicine discovered their properties. It is believed that two-thirds of the world's plant species have some medicinal importance and that almost all of them have antioxidant properties [277]. This makes sense, considering that plants are constantly assaulted by oxidative agents and need robust defensive mechanisms. They are bombarded by high-energy UV light rays, which convert carbon dioxide into highly reactive oxygen. Without antioxidants, plants wouldn't survive the very same process that gives them the energy to grow.

Oriental Herbs

In 2002, it was estimated that over 50,000 medicinal plants were in used and traded commercially in common markets [278]. That number has likely grown since then, given the recent interest in cheaper forms of treatment and the widespread adoption of online shopping. With so many plants to cover, it would be impossible to cover them all in this book. Considering that antioxidant properties are universal to almost all plants, it's likely that a vast majority of the 50,000 medicinal plants that are in use today will have *some* positive effect on acne. Even so, let's take a look at some of the most promising plants.

Chinese goldthread *(Coptis Chinensis)* was found to reduce sebum production when applied to the skin [279]. Similar to barberries, this plant is rich in the berberine compound, which explains the acne-fighting abilities. This plant's sebum-suppressing effect was even more potent than that of retinoic acid, another common commercial treatment for acne. Similar positive results were found in *sea buckthorn* [280]*, saw palmetto, sesame seeds, and argan oil* [281].

Dahurian Angelica (Angelica Dahurica) has been found to have anti-inflammatory properties by preventing the migration of white blood cells to the site of injury [282]. Cells that come into contact with foreign pathogens emit signaling chemicals, named *chemotactic factors,* that direct white blood cells to where they are needed. If you prevent the production of chemotactic factors, then you also disable the navigation system of white blood cells, thus avoiding inflammation [283]. The Dahurian Angelica plant was found to stop this migration of white blood cells to skin regions that come into contact with the C. acnes bacteria. This effect was found to be just as powerful as erythromycin – a commercial anti-inflammatory drug [282]. Similar anti-inflammatory properties were found in the following plants: *Abies koreana* [284], *Aralia continentalis* [285], *Clerodendrum trichotomum* [286], *Coptis chinensis* [287], *Echinacea purpurea* [288], *Eucommia ulmoides Oliv* [289], *Garcinia mangostana* [290], *Ilex paraguariensis* [289], *Magnolia sp.* [291], *Punica granatum* [292], *Selaginella involvens* [293], *Camellia sinensis L.* [294], and many others [295].

Licorice (Glycyrrhiza glabra) has been shown to have antimicrobial properties against colonies of C. acnes, comparable to the commercial drug *erythromycin*. What's more, the bacteria treated with licorice didn't develop resistance, unlike the colonies treated with erythromycin. This indicates that licorice might be a better long-term treatment against acne, as bacteria don't become as immune to the treatment [282]. Mind you, the test was done in-vitro by applying extracts of this plant directly on the bacteria. Similar to green tea extracts, to get the full range of antimicrobial properties, one would have to apply lotions of licorice on the skin instead of eating it straight up. Other plants shown to have antimicrobial properties include *Butyrospermum paradoxicum* [296], *Commiphora mukul* [297], *Melaleuca alternifolia* [298], *Ocimum basilicum* [297], *Ocimum gratissimum* [299], and many others [295].

A lotion consisting of **Leuns culinaris**, **Aloe barbadensis**, **Vitex negundo**, **Arographis paniculate,** and **Salmalia malabaric** was administered to 26 acne-sufferers for a trial period of six weeks. After just two weeks into the experiment, there was a significant reduction in the number of blackheads and whiteheads compared to the start of the trial [300]. This mixture was reported to have antimicrobial, anti-inflammatory, and sex-hormone suppressing effects. The last property – the ability to stop the production of sex hormones – hasn't been discussed so far, but it is an important risk factor for acne that will get its own chapter later in the book. Until then, we'll just mention that similar properties were found in other plants as well, including *Serenoa repens, Sesamum indicum, Argania spinosa* [301].

As you can see, it's entirely possible to target almost all risk factors of acne using just plant-based medicine. Some of the natural treatments have passed modern scientific rigor. More so, several such plants are more effective and have fewer side effects compared to their commercial counterparts. Still, not all traditional medicine has been proven to work, and some might even be detrimental to our health. It's essential to research any alternative treatment before investing your time, money, and health.

If researching alternative plants is too much effort, then green tea remains one of the cheapest and well-studied forms of acne treatment, and you can't go wrong by trying it. It interacts with almost all risk factors for this disease, including inflammation, sebum production, cell proliferation, and bacterial growth. Green tea should still be your number one choice if you're considering treating acne without changing your diet. Chances are, you're already drinking tea without knowing it has so many beneficial effects.

CHAPTER SUMMARY

- In-vitro tests have shown that green tea prevents inflammation, kills the acne-causing bacteria, and suppresses several acne-inducing transcription factors. Most laboratory tests on samples of skin cells indicate that green tea is an effective treatment against acne.

- Interventional experiments confirmed the positive results of green tea. Acne patients that were given green tea saw a reduction in pimple count and a general improvement in acne conditions.

- Other plants have shown similar positive effects against acne. Some traditional oriental herbs can reduce inflammation, kill the C. acnes bacteria, decrease sex hormones production, and reduce sebum flow. However, green tea remains the most researched plant and is considerably easier to come by and cheaper compared to the alternatives.

ALCOHOL

Not long ago, it was common practice for doctors and nurses to go from the autopsy room straight into surgery, without so much as a simple washing of hands. Back then, mortality rates in hospitals were high, especially for newborns and their mothers. As early as the mid 19th century, one in every five newborns would die from mysterious fevers caught in the hospital. Although it's inconceivable to us nowadays how doctors could handle cadavers in one moment and live patients the next, that's how medicine operated for most of humanity's history. Back then, we didn't know about germs and viruses, and we had a minimal understanding of how diseases spread. There was little incentive for medical practitioners to stay clean and keep their hands sanitary, which is why mortality rates were so high in hospitals during the previous centuries.

It took one pioneer, named Ignaz Semmelweis, to change this and revolutionize the way we think about hospital cleanliness. Semmelweis observed that infant mortality rates were much higher in certain clinics than in others, and he set out to understand why.

Semmelweis also observed that doctors and medical students often went into the delivery room after performing autopsies with considerable odors on their hands [302]. His theory was that this odor was caused by "cadaverous particles" that were transmitted from the dead bodies to the newborns via the doctors' unwashed hands. He then proposed that all medical practitioners first wash their hands with a chlorinates lime solution after each autopsy to dissolve the fever-carrying particles. Once these health measures were implemented, infant mortality rates plummeted, falling from 16% to 3% on average.

We now know that the "cadaverous particles" were infectious microorganisms, too small to be visible to the naked eye, but which can easily be transmitted through our hands. The first germs of this kind were discovered as late as the 1890s [303], which only became possible with the invention of the microscope. This discovery came quite late in the timeline of medical advancements, considering that the first vaccine was invented some 200 years earlier [304].

Today, we have a pretty good grasp on what causes infectious diseases and how to prevent them. With the recent COVID-19 epidemic, the general population has become even more educated on how to prevent the spread of such illnesses, using a combination of hand sanitizers, frequent hand washing, masks, and physical distancing. Alcohol itself has become indispensable to the way we prevent diseases, either by using it as a disinfectant on fresh wounds or by periodically sanitizing our hands using a quick splash of hand cleansers. No medicine cabinet is complete without it.

Given our modern understanding of how alcohols prevent bacteria and viruses from spreading, it's natural to assume that this sanitizer can also help prevent acne. Because pimples form when bacteria seep deep within our skin, if you kill off the bacteria, you also prevent the release of pro-inflammatory signaling proteins that promote the growth of inflamed pimples. This is how certain acne medications work – such as benzoyl peroxide and tea tree extracts. They kill the bacteria on our skin before it gets a chance to penetrate skin pores. Even if a pore blockage does occur, there's less chance of it becoming inflamed if no bacteria are present. Seeing as alcohols have similar antibacterial properties to benzoyl peroxide and other topical acne treatments, we should expect them to have positive effects on our skin.

And we would be right; alcohol does kill the acne-promoting bacteria, as well as many other different types of microscopic pathogens. But this comes with a catch. Many substances can kill bacteria in a petri dish, including cyanide and sulphuric acid. The problem with these antibacterial substances is that they also kill healthy cells as well.

By definition, for a substance to be considered an "alcohol," it must possess a water-loving molecule called a *hydroxyl*. This end of the alcohol compound is electrically charged and allows the entire molecule to interact well with water and other water-loving chemicals, including the membrane of most cells.

The water-loving part of the alcohol molecule interacts with the outer layer of a cell membrane, disrupting its structure [305]. If sufficient alcohol is present around a cell, it completely dissolves the protective membrane, spewing the cell's innards. As you can imagine, this has a terminal effect on the cell, killing it altogether.

This is why alcohol is so effective at killing bacteria and viruses. All bacterial cells and some viruses are protected by an outer membrane that is dissolved by alcohol compounds. If you expose these pathogens to alcohols, the protective outer layer breaks down, spilling the guts outwards, killing them completely. However, this cell-killing effect doesn't happen only for foreign pathogens but for all types of cells which have the same protective membrane – including healthy human cells.

If you apply alcohol to human cells, then they can die off as well. Although human skin has some protection against environmental damage, the defenses can't last forever. If you apply alcohol long enough on the skin, you will start to damage living skin cells, leading to dryness, irritation, and redness.

What's more, alcohols have one more property that makes them especially dangerous to our skin. They have high permeability, allowing them to penetrate deeper into our skin compared to other chemicals. Because of this, the damage brought by alcohol is not superficial but can affect living cells from deeper within our skin. The high permeability of alcohols is also the reason why they are so popular with cosmetic and dermatologic products – they act as a Trojan Horse, carrying the active ingredients from these products into our skin.

Once inside our skin, besides the direct damage to skin cell membranes, alcohols also directly stimulate the production of pro-inflammatory signaling proteins. Experiments have shown that human skin cells exposed to ethanol (the type of alcohol found in alcoholic beverages) released pro-inflammatory proteins, potentially causing swelling and redness to the affected area [306]. The study showed that this toxic effect is visible even in low ethanol concentrations, far smaller than what we would typically find in cosmetic products.

All of this means that the damaging effect on skin cells outweighs any benefits brought by the antimicrobial properties of alcohols. Simply put, other topical acne treatments work better and have fewer side effects, so there's no point in risking our health when we have far safer alternatives. Yes, the temptation is high as alcohols are much cheaper and easier to come by than other acne treatments. But this is one temptation we should fight strongly.

Because alcohols are so damaging to healthy cells, there haven't been any experiments that test alcohol lotions as a potential treatment against acne. For the most part, we can rule out alcohol as a topical treatment against acne. However, we have other ways to use alcohol that are a lot more fun than irritating our skin: drinking it as a beverage.

There have been plenty of epidemiological studies that link alcohol consumption with acne, but they don't all agree with one another. For example, one research performed in Korea found that alcohol consumption was associated with an increased risk of developing acne [307], while another study conducted in Lithuania showed no such association [308].

It should be noted that the average age range of the two studies was quite different, which could have affected the results. The research in Korea included people of all ages, while the one from

Lithuania only included adolescents aged 7 to 19. There's more incentive for children and young adults to lie about their alcohol drinking habits, considering that drinking alcohol at such a young age is frowned upon, and illegal in most places. Thus, the difference between the two studies can simply be attributed to the reliability of answers from the participants.

More so, during adolescence, other risk factors can cause acne and outweigh the effects of alcohol. This topic will be explored at length in the

Puberty and Hormones chapter. Still, for now, it's enough to know that the bodily changes that occur during this period of development can also influence our skin to make us more prone to breaking out. Alcohol, it seems, can interfere with this process, changing not only how well we go through these transitional phases but also how likely we are to get pimples.

*

During the early stages of our life, several internal organs emit signals that direct the human body to transform into fully functioning adults. I'm sure you're well aware of the changes that go on in our bodies during childhood and adolescence. We grow in stature, in mass, our voice deepens, and sex-specific organs develop to maturity. These transformations are driven by signals emitted either from the brain directly or through auxiliary organs specific to each sex.

Besides body growth and transformation, I'm sure you've also noticed that acne is much more common during adolescence compared to any other period of our life. This explosion in acne cases is caused by a mixup of signals between our skin and other organs meant to grow and develop during this time. The same messages that direct the body to transform into adults will also trigger our skin to produce more sebum and generally promote acne [309].

It might seem that pubertal acne is unavoidable, seeing as we wouldn't want to interfere with the normal growth and development changes that occur in our body during this time. However, this is not entirely true, as some of these signals can be amplified to dangerous levels by factors that are under our control and which we abuse regularly. Only some nations experience high acne rates during adolescence [1], even though the genetic makeup is almost identical between all of us. This has lead researchers to speculate that the acne we get while growing up is still caused by human-made factors.

Several aspects can interfere with the growth and development signals emitted during puberty. We will get the complete list in the

Puberty and Hormones chapter, but it seems that alcohol can also manipulate these messages that harm our skin.

During puberty, the human body emits two broad signals that direct the entire ensemble to mature: a growth signal that causes organs to grow in size, and a sex-differentiation signal that promotes the formation of male or female-specific traits. This information is transmitted throughout our body using hormones, which are nothing more than chemical couriers that carry a message from one part of the body to another. These hormones can be emitted either directly by our brain through special glands located at its base or by other organs, including the liver, pancreas, and even stomach.

It is now believed that both hormone classes (growth and sex-differentiation) can exacerbate acne by interfering with the three major acne-related transcription factors: mTOR, FoxOs, and SREBPs. Some hormones are more potent than others at promoting acne, and their production can be influenced by the alcohol that we drink.

Take, for example, IGF-1, a growth-stimulating hormone that is secreted abundantly during early childhood. Previously, we also saw that excessive levels of IGF-1 could cause acne by interfering with several transcription factors that control sebum production, inflammation, and bacterial growth [160]. Milk and dairy products stimulate the production of IGF-1 through their high-protein content [310], which makes this food group especially dangerous to our skin.

Recent evidence suggests that alcohol consumption can also interfere with this process, but by having the exact opposite effect to milk. It was found that moderate alcohol consumption can potentially improve acne conditions by suppressing the production of IGF-1 [311].

The liver is the main organ where IGF-1 is made. Thus, one would expect that foods or drinks that disturb the liver's normal functioning can also affect the production of IGF-1. Alcohol is a famous example of such a substance that interferes with the liver.

In the short term, drinking large amounts of alcohol – even for just a few days – can lead to a buildup of fat deposits in the liver [312]. The liver typically clears itself out after a few weeks of abstinence from alcohol, but chronic alcohol consumption will prevent the liver from healing itself in the long run. If fat deposits continue to build up in the liver, it can eventually lead to complications such as liver fibrosis or even cancer [313].

Recent experiments have shown that even moderate alcohol consumption can lead to short-term hormonal changes in the body due to alcohol's interaction with the liver. In one such experiment, eight patients were asked to drink a diluted form of ethanol (the type of alcohol found in alcoholic beverages), equivalent to only 2% of a glass of regular beer. After 3 hours of drinking the alcoholic beverages, blood levels of IGF-1 were measured and compared to samples taken before the drinking session.

Researchers found that IGF-1 levels decreased by 13% in people who drank alcoholic beverages [311]. These low levels of IGF-1 were found even after a full night's sleep by the participants. Seeing as these effects were observed after consuming just 1/50th of a glass of beer, a regular drinking session will likely cause even larger drops in circulating IGF-1 levels.

Since IGF-1 production decreases after drinking a glass of an alcoholic beverage, one would expect that regular alcohol consumption will be protective against acne. However, real-world data isn't very conclusive. At the beginning of this chapter, we saw that studies that analyze the drinking habits of ordinary people find that alcohol is neutral in some and even worsens acne in others. It's clear that the interaction with IGF-1 is not enough to explain alcohol's influence on our skin.

These conflictual results can likely be explained by the fact that alcohol's protective effects don't last very long. IGF-1 levels recover after 1 to 2 days of consuming an alcoholic beverage. More so, besides interfering with the liver's normal function, alcohols also interact with other hormones that exacerbate acne, canceling these probable protective effects.

*

During puberty, besides growth hormones, the human body also emits hormones that direct the body to develop gender-specific characteristics. This includes the reproductive organs themselves, but also organs that are considered "secondary sex characteristics," such as the excess hair growth we see in our pubic area, armpits, and face.

Although the basic sex organs are present at birth, they don't become fully functional until mid to late adolescence. We all remember the awkward moments from our youths when our bodies began to change in unexpected and usually embarrassing ways. Extra hair growth, menstruation, erections, the deepening of the voice – they all happen because our body emits sex hormones that direct some organs to develop fully.

Several hormones stimulate the development of female organs, like breasts and the uterus. Other hormones trigger the maturation of male organs, such as the penis or testicles. Some sex hormones are present in both men and women, causing the development of sex characteristics common to both sexes. For example, hair growth near the genitals happens for both genders and is activated by sex hormones common to men and women. What's more, the hormones that cause hair growth also drive sebum secretion equally in all genders [160] [314].

Because sex hormones play such a crucial role in hair maturation and skin health, they are also a cornerstone of our understanding of how acne forms. Again, we will explore this topic at length in the

Puberty and Hormones chapter, but for now, it's enough to mention that only the male sex hormones stimulate sebum production. However, this does not mean that only men can get acne. In fact, women are more likely to have acne compared to men [315]. The reason why both genders can have acne is due to some unique proteins that can convert from one form of sex hormone to another.

Not all sex hormones are equally potent. Some stimulate sebum production more than others. Some hormones are relatively inert, and they barely register as sex-differentiation signals. Others are incredibly potent and can cause large amounts of sebum production. Testosterone is one famous hormone from this class, responsible for supporting male sex organs and driving sebum production. However, other hormones are ten times more potent than testosterone and pose a bigger threat to our skin [316].

The human body can convert from one type of hormone to another through specialized enzymes that act as catalysts to this transformation process. Unlucky for us, our skin contains all necessary enzymes that can convert from relatively inert forms of male sex hormones to the most potent ones.

Both women and men have these enzymes, which is why women can still have large amounts of what we consider male sex hormones without developing actual male organs. Human skin cells can convert harmless forms of sex hormones into testosterone and other sebum-producing hormones. To prevent pimples, it's much more important to control this conversion process rather than stopping sex hormones altogether.

Certain factors can interfere with this conversion process. Some signals can cause skin cells to produce more sex hormones, while others stop the production altogether. It seems that alcohol is one such factor that stimulates the production of sebum-producing hormones.

Experiments have shown that ethanol, when applied directly to cells, activates the enzyme that converts testosterone into more powerful hormones [317]. In turn, these hormones boost the production of sebum much more compared to simple testosterone [318]. This increase in sebum production can lead to blocked pores and eventually acne. Admittedly, this effect was observed only in rat cells and only for organs that come into direct contact with alcoholic beverages (mouth, throat, and esophagus). However, we have no reason to believe that these results don't apply to humans as well.

It's also important to stress that sex hormones are not present only during puberty but stay with us throughout our life – albeit in significantly fewer quantities. Alcohol can still interfere with the normal function of these hormones well into our adult years, making us more prone to breakouts even after our sex organs develop fully.

Besides stimulating the hormone conversion process, it seems that alcohol also encourages the production of testosterone itself. Multiple experiments have shown that consuming even low dosages of alcoholic beverages can increase the blood circulating levels of testosterone [319] [320]. However, this effect is not major, and it's unlikely to impact acne significantly. Still, considering that testosterone promotes aggression in male individuals, the alcohol-driven increase in testosterone has led some scientists to believe that this effect explains why some people exhibit more aggressive behavior after a few drinks [321].

Overall, alcohol consumption has mixed effects on acne. On the one hand, alcohol decreases the production of IGF-1 – a known acne-inducing hormone – thus having a protective effect on our skin. But it also stimulates the production of certain sex hormones that are thought to aggravate acne.

The net effect points towards alcohol being relatively harmless to our skin, so you can likely continue having an occasional drink and not worry about breaking out. Despite this, alcohol consumption has other known negative influences on our health, including increasing our risk of developing heart disease, stroke, liver disease, and various cancers. In addition, excessive alcohol consumption is also known to weaken our immune system, create cognitive problems, social phobias [322], and promote some other 60 different types of diseases and conditions [323].

Because alcohol is such a threat to our health, most nations have introduced a tax on alcoholic beverages to discourage their consumption. Similarly, some countries have banned alcoholic beverages altogether (although this is usually done due to religious reasons rather than health concerns). Your risk of dying rises for as little as one glass of wine per day, especially for men [324]. Even if alcohol and acne are not strongly linked, you should still avoid drinking alcoholic beverages as much as possible to prevent developing other, more severe health problems.

CHAPTER SUMMARY

- Alcohol-based skin disinfectants work by breaking down the outer membrane of germs, spilling the innards, thus killing the pathogens. Alcohol can also kill acne-promoting bacteria through the same mechanism.

- Although alcohol kills the bacteria that cause acne, it also kills healthy skin cells. This can cause skin irritation and inflammation, potentially making acne even worse. For this reason, alcohol should not be used as a topical treatment against acne, considering there are other options that work better and have fewer side effects.

- Drinking alcoholic beverages is likely safe and doesn't aggravate acne. On the one hand, alcohol consumption has been shown to decrease blood levels of IGF-1, thus having a protective effect. However, alcohol also increases the production of certain sex hormones, which are through to exacerbate acne. Overall, alcohol seems to be neutral to our skin, making it safe for occasional consumption.

SALT

Imagine being an infinitesimally small spec inside an immense glass cloud, one that spans the entire known universe and is several million million million times the diameter of our Solar system. If the cloud were perfectly symmetrical, it would stay this way indefinitely, eventually cooling and expanding into a cold, empty, and dead glob of nothingness. But the cloud is not symmetrical. It has slight bumps and clumps that put gravity at work to twist and morph the entire mass of primordial soup into much more interesting shapes – albeit very slowly. If you wait long enough, fine particles of gas start sticking to each other, forming flat discs of cloud that spin quickly into a uniform direction. You're in one such disc, but you would never know, as everything is still so stretched apart that at your scale, nothing seems to be moving.

But gravity never stops and continues to pull *everything* deeper within the disc. And there's only so much space that you can fit stuff into. Even if everything started as a dispersed cloud of almost nothing, as you squeeze the fine particles closer and closer together, they starting bumping into each other more violently with each passing moment.

You start speeding up. All the accumulated energy from the dispersed gas cloud has to go somewhere and is transferred into the motion of particles that make up the immense disc. Everything around you becomes more chaotic and violent as mater is brought closer together. The mist of particles, although only a fraction in size compared to the initial gas giant, is still several thousand times bigger and several thousand times heavier than our Solar system. There's nothing in the human experience to compare this process to. The scale is so large, and everything moves so slowly that nothing noticeable would change in the course of a single human life.

It's not long until fine gas molecules start whizzing about so quickly that they emit light. You start seeing faint hues of red sparks, almost like an aurora but permeated through everything around you. As pressure and temperature continue to build up, the light around you becomes brighter and turns to every color of the rainbow; first to orange, then yellow, and finally to pure white. But the light around you is no longer emitted because everything is extremely hot. Instead, particles smash into each other with such force that it disintegrates matter itself to make pure energy. Gravity has finally found its match. It can no longer squeeze gas clumps into smaller spaces, as it's counteracted by a much greater force, fueled by matter itself. But this victory doesn't last long. Gravity never stops.

Each time you smash into other particles, you fuse together, becoming undisguisable with each transformation. You become heavier. It takes a lot more force to move you around. If the initial gas cloud were light enough, you would continue emitting energy into the nothingness of space until you cool down to become an invisible ball of cool rock that can't be seen even with the most powerful of telescopes. But that's not the case for you. The stuff around you is just heavy enough to allow gravity to continue its march. You're squeezed even harder. Pressure builds up until... catastrophe. The forces around you are so extreme that matter goes through one final transformation, one that releases so much energy that everything around you explodes with an immense shockwave. In a split second, this explosion releases 100 times more energy than our Sun will radiate throughout its 10 billion-year lifespan. This eruption is so forceful that it smashes you into other particles with such intensity that it changes your very core chemical fabric.

You're blasted into empty space with a speed so high that it would take you only 15 seconds to traverse the distance between Earth and our Moon. For some time, you exist in suspension in the nothingness of space, all alone. But gravity never stops.

You and the specks that were thrown off from the initial exposition start clumping together again. But this time, you're luckier. There's not enough stuff to help gravity do its full dance. This time, you do get squeezed with other particles into a big ball of matter, but one which is allowed to cool and take a stable round shape. As the bubble you're in cools and is crumpled together by gravity, it solidifies with a hard shell of rock. But don't be fooled. Even if the outer shell gives appearances of serenity and stability, the center still remains hot, liquid, and forever moving. Although the pressure inside this ball is much less than that of the initial gas cloud, it's still large enough to force the hot liquid into one final explosion. You get pushed again through small cracks of the hard outer shell, dissolving any minerals that come into contact with you. Eventually, you reach water and get absorbed. You're unrecognizable from your initial self.

But your journey is not over yet.

As water starts to evaporate, you emerge into a shimmering crystal, one with a shape that is defined by the very fabric that holds you together. You and the other atoms left behind from water's departure start sticking together into a predefined ensemble dictated by Mother Nature itself. One by one, you start building scaffolding for what will eventually become a microscopic cube, born in chaos but culminated as a perfect geometrical shape. You sparkle pure white light, making you resemble a nobler grain of sand.

You get scooped up one last time.

After a journey of billions of years, being squeezed, exploded, disjointed, dissolved, and evaporated, your final resting place is... on someone's enchiladas.

That's right; you're table salt.

Ordinary table salt had an extraordinary journey to reach your kitchen top. Although salt is very chemically simple with just two atoms, the process of creating them was extremely lengthy and required an enormous amount of energy. We don't think twice about the nature and history of salt when we add it to our food, even though it's the most consumed food condiment in the world.

Annually, we consume over 300 million metric tons of salt [325]. Because it is used in nearly every dish that we eat, it has been the target for fortification with essential nutrients (such as iodine) by most countries of the world. Yet, despite salt's popularity as a food condiment, it also has a bad reputation when it comes to health.

It's commonly cited as increasing the risk of heart disease – the leading cause of death in westernized countries. The World Health Organization estimates that up to 2.5 million people die each year due to excessive sodium consumption, which mostly comes from the extra salt we eat in processed food and items prepared outside the home [326]. The reason why salt has this negative influence on our health comes down to how the constituents of salt are used by our body to maintain optimal fluid levels and how excess salt consumption cripples this system. This very same imbalance that leads to high blood pressure and other related complications is also why excess salt consumption is believed to worsen acne.

As you might know from elementary chemistry lessons, common table salt is comprised of just two major chemicals: sodium and chloride. Both of these chemicals are essential to human health and help keep the optimal fluid level outside and inside our cells. Too little of either chemical is dangerous to our health, but too much can be equally damaging. In salt-loving Western nations, it's much more common to have a surplus of sodium and chloride in our diet, leading to a fluid imbalance in our body.

Water is an essential substance for all known living creatures, including humans. It is used everywhere from temperature regulation, nutrient transport, digestion, waste removal, protection of various organs, and many other roles. Because it's so crucial to life, the human body has evolved several ways to regulate it and to maintain optimal fluid levels throughout our body.

One might think that cells have tiny pumps that push water in and out as needed. But most living organisms have evolved a much more ingenious way to regulate fluid levels without needing so much energy. In fact, our cells don't need any energy at all, only salt.

Water is present in most human tissue, including our blood, most living cells, and the space between them (aptly named the extra-cellular fluid). When our cells need additional fluids, they draw extra water from the area around them. Too much water in our cells, and they swell up and burst. Too little water, and they shrivel and die. Maintaining the right balance of fluid in our cells is vital to their health.

Pumping water in and out of cells would require enormous amounts of energy if it were done actively through a pump. Running such a small pump for each and every cell in our body would eat up just too many precious nutrients to be viable. Instead, Mother Nature, being ingenious as always, uses a property of fluids that contain dissolved salts to cleverly move liquids around without any energy. This process is called *osmosis,* and it's also one technique we use to purify drinking water. We discovered this property only a few hundred years ago, but Mother Nature has been using osmosis to power life for billions of years.

You might remember from high school physics lessons that when we say that some substance has a certain temperature, we are actually describing the average speed of all molecules that make up that substance. The higher the temperature, the faster the molecules whizz around. This happens for all mediums, be it solids, fluids, or gases. If it has a positive absolute temperature, then the molecules are jiggling about and smashing into each other.

This jiggling happens in water molecules as well. If a medium is liquid and has a positive temperature, then the motion of the molecules will cause them to move constantly. The higher the temperature, the faster the movement. This is why, If you allow enough time, water-based solutions will eventually mix into a homogenous blend if placed next to each other. For example, if you add a small drop of ink into a glass of water, the entire solution eventually turns light purple. Because both the water and the ink molecules have a positive temperature and are constantly whizzing about, they will ultimately blend into a uniform solution.

The same process happens with the water inside us. The fluid in our body is warm enough to encourage the movement of water molecules and any dissolved nutrients. This property of warm liquids can be used to transport useful products within and outside a cell. Water can transport nutrients through a cell membrane, but it can also move waste products outside a cell.

However, this property of liquids is not enough to create a fully functioning transportation highway. You still need to control the direction of this movement. You wouldn't want to pump nutrients out of a healthy cell, similar to how you wouldn't want to inject waste products inside a cell.

The trick is to add minerals to one side of a cell membrane, such that it blocks the movement of water from that direction. Instead of moving freely in and outside a cell, water molecules will now smash into these barriers and not be allowed to pass through. These minerals act as a one-way valve, allowing the movement of fluids only to the space that has fewer dissolved salts. This is precisely the role sodium and chloride play. They act as barriers that allow fluids to move from one side of a cell membrane but not the other. By adding more or fewer salts inside or outside of a cell, you can direct the flow of water and, with it, nutrients.

If the human body lacks sufficient sodium or chloride salts (also called electrolytes), then cells lose the ability to regulate fluid levels. However, the reverse can be just as bad. If our body has too many electrolytes, this can cause a local buildup of fluid needed to maintain optimal concentrations of salts in our blood and our cells. When this happens, human tissue swells in size. Sometimes, this has a visible and often painful effect. Most of us have had swollen feet or hands at some point in our life, which was likely caused by fluid buildup in the affected area.

This excess fluid retention can also happen in our skin, including the skin from our face. Diets high in salt that cause a buildup of sodium and chloride in the extra-cellular fluid will also cause water retention and swelling throughout our body. This swelling can also cause skin pores to be constricted, preventing the normal flow of sebum. As sebum pressure builds inside these tightened skin pores, the pressure can become so large that the skin ruptures, leading to inflammation and pimples. This is the reason why some suspect salty foods cause acne. If you eat excess salt and sodium, it can cause a buildup of fluid in the skin, leading to limited sebum flow and potentially acne.

However, this effect remains purely hypothetical, as there haven't been that many studies on this topic. In reality, the amount of fluid retention in the face caused by eating excess salt is likely too small to have any noticeable effect on our skin. Even so, one study performed in 2016 found that people who eat salty foods do tend to have more acne than average. The sample was quite small, with only 200 respondents. But, even in this small group of people, the researchers found that acne patients go over the recommended daily limit of salt more often than clear-skin individuals. On average, 76% of people with acne go over the recommended limit for salt, compared to just 46% for the general population. Even the patients themselves believed that salt was the cause of their acne; 34% of acne patients reported increases in acne lesions after eating salty foods [327].

Another study on the link between sodium intake and acne was performed all the way back in 1965. The experiment was set up as an interventional study in which a medical practitioner suggested various dietary changes to his acne patients. For some patients, the physician suggested reducing sodium intake for a few days to see if their acne condition improves. By the end of the experiment, four of the patients that were asked to drop salt saw a noticeable improvement in their skin [328].

Although these might seem like promising results, when we consider that only 30 patients participated in the no-salt challenge, we can see that the success rate is pretty low, at only 13% - much lower than other acne treatments. What's more, this experiment also lacked a placebo group, meaning that the patients likely improved just by pure chance rather than due to the dietary changes.

Overall, there is no concrete evidence to suggest that consuming normal quantities of salt has any effect on acne. However, there's no harm in reducing sodium intake for a short experiment to see if this change does help with your acne. If nothing else, keeping circulating sodium levels within recommended levels can have other health benefits, including a lower chance of dying from heart disease [329] [330] and improvements in edema conditions [331]. Even so, if you are planning on experimenting with dietary changes, I wouldn't start with salt, but with some other food items which have a much stronger association with acne, like dairy and high-protein foods.

CHAPTER SUMMARY

- The sodium and chloride found in salt are critical to the normal function of almost all human cells, as they help regulate fluid levels in and outside cells.

- Too much salt intake can cause water retention and swelling. If this happens in the skin, it can constrict skin pores, blocking the normal flow of sebum and increasing the chances of pimples forming.

- Although swelling due to excess salt does happen in our skin, it usually happens in our feet and hands rather than the face. To date, there have been no strong studies that suggest that high salt intake has any measurable effect on acne.

Part II

LIFESTYLE & ENVIRONMENT

STOP TOUCHING YOUR FACE!

There are many aspects of acne that make it not only a stigmatizing and embarrassing disease but also one which causes a lot of frustration for those affected. Intuitively, it seems like an easy problem to fix. Because acne is formed when skin pores become clogged with gunk, if we were to wash our face more often to eliminate all this junk, then we would also improve acne. Because of this, acne appears, for most, a problem of personal hygiene rather than a "real disease."

But, after reading this book, you should by now see that this idea that acne is caused by personal hygiene is far from the truth. Yet, this myth remains, causing frustration for those that suffer from this disease. That's not to say that acne doesn't have *some* hygiene component to it – we will take the rest of the chapter to find out if this is true. Rather, all the research made on this topic so far and which was explored in this book puts diet and not hygiene at the top of the list of acne-causing factors.

At the end of the day, acne is a complicated disease that we don't fully understand yet. Trivializing it by blaming it all on hygiene will only prevent those affected from getting real help that actually works. Even more, some experiments have shown that over-washing can be detrimental to our skin, exacerbating acne even more [332]. This misconception that acne is primarily caused by a lack of cleanliness will not only prevent sufferers from getting the treatment they need but might also make the problem worse.

The fact that most people are not aware of the many contributing factors for acne is one reason why it can be frustrating for sufferers to deal with this disease. Although well-intentioned, most of the advice we hear from friends and family will likely not help in the slightest, amplifying the despair some of us have even more.

The most common advice, "Stop touching your face," is one that has a negligible effect on acne and is repeated often. The fact that we have to constantly watch our hand movements and be aware of everything that touches our faces will amplify the stress we feel from this disease. When, inevitably, these tactics don't show signs of working, we will likely default to blaming ourselves as we didn't take sufficient care of our face. It's no wonder then that acne sufferers have significantly higher depression rates than average [333].

The fact that personal hygiene is a commonly cited root cause of acne can cause clear-skin people to perceive acne sufferers as dirty and greasy. This can only amplify the social stigma some acne patients feel when interacting with other people, thus leading to long-lasting social phobias [334]. This is why we must understand the real causes of acne and educate those around us. We shouldn't blame ourselves for getting pimples, and we should especially not blame our hygiene for this condition. Acne is an extremely complicated disease, one that can take up to 12 weeks to improve once we make the appropriate changes in our lifestyle [335].

So far in this book, we've explored mostly dietary factors that can contribute to acne. We've seen that certain foods increase the likelihood of developing pimples, either by increasing the rate of sebum production, changing the viscosity of sebum, increasing the rate at which skin cells die, or which put our immune system into overdrive. Some of these foods can affect many or all of these factors.

But, so far, we haven't looked at some of the more mechanical aspects of acne. We know the basics of how pimples form, but to get a complete picture of how everything works and how to prevent acne, we must also understand what happens at a microscopic level. Through this learning process, we will be able to finally confirm or dispel the myth that a lack of hygiene is the main factor that can lead to acne.

How pimples form

Most people are aware that sebum, an oily substance secreted by our skin, is heavily implicated in acne formation. The function of this substance is to protect our skin from foreign microorganisms and help with temperature control. It has these properties because sebum is, in reality, a mixture of multiple ingredients, some of them being used for lubrication and temperature control, while others are slightly acidic and help kill harmful pathogens.

One of these acids, called *sapienic acid*, is unique to humans and is a major component of human sebum. This molecule provides the anti-bacterial properties of sebum and is vital in fighting off the bacteria that cause acne. The oily bits in sebum helps keep the entire mixture glued to the skin, while the acidic part destroys microbes before they can inflict further damage. Because of this, sebum is important to the health of our skin. It helps prevent an overgrowth of bacteria and viruses that can cause infection or other diseases.

If you stop the production of sebum, then you risk developing complications from the lack of a protective film, leading to dry skin and irritation [336]. This is precisely what happens with certain acne medications, like isotretinoin, whose primary mechanism of action is to stop sebum flow altogether. Although these medications help prevent acne by stopping the production of sebum, they also lead to severe side effects caused by a lack of a protective layer on our skin. Because of this, when fighting acne, we don't want to completely stop the production of sebum. Instead, we want to maintain both the flow and the composition at optimal levels, such that we don't get pimples, and we also keep the protective mantle.

Our body needs a way to pump this mixture onto our skin, but in a way that distributes everything evenly across the surface. Instead of creating new injection places, the human body has evolved to re-use the existing chamber through which hairs poke through. By re-using these pores, sebum can also lubricate the hair itself, which helps maintain a stable body temperature.

It is more evident in men rather than in women, but our entire skin is covered with tiny hairs, including our foreheads, cheeks, arms, and legs. Small glands that continuously produce sebum are positioned at the base of these hairs. As there's no place for this mixture to go other than up, once enough sebum is made, it is squeezed up the hair follicle to reach the outer skin surface. All of these components are summarized in *Figure 16*.

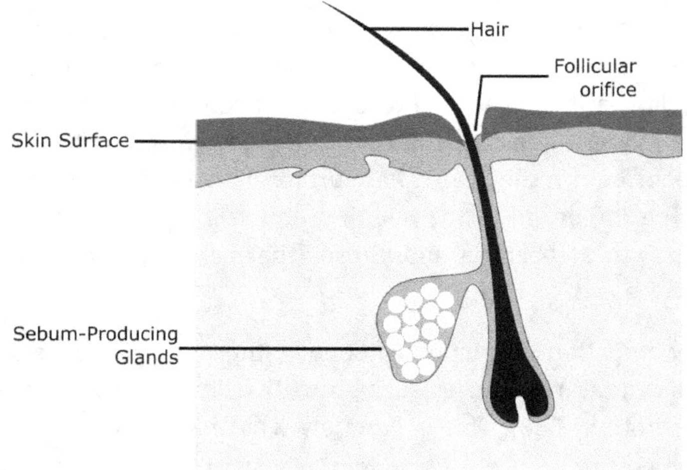

Figure 16 - Normal hair follicle

These glands do not directly produce sebum. Instead, they incubate tiny cells – called sebocytes – which act as small balloons that are gradually filled with all of the ingredients needed to make this oily substance.

After an incubation period of around 14-20 days, these cells fill up to the point of bursting, spilling the inner mixture inside the sebum-producing glands. This means that these glands don't release just sebum but also a series of dead skin cells that nurtured sebum to maturity. The ratio between the two will affect the stickiness and viscosity of the resulting mixture. If the proportion is out of balance, sebum will flow much harder out the hair chambers. Similarly, if the mixture reaches a specific thickness, it will stop flowing completely, creating blockages and pimples.

Both sebum and the dead skin cells are created deep within the hair chambers that are situated inside our skin. When the conditions are right, and this mix of sebum and skin cells becomes too viscous to flow efficiently out the pore, then a blockage occurs, and a pimple is formed.

This means that acne is an inside-out process. The ingredients needed to produce these blockages are created within the skin, where dirt and other external materials can't easily get in. All of the pimple-causing elements are self-contained within our hair chambers. The outer gunk that might be found on our skin has minimal contribution to the entire process.

As we've already talked about in the first part of this book, many factors can affect sebum's viscosity.

On the one hand, sebum quality is dependent on essential fatty acids levels, which includes linoleic acid. Similarly, certain saturated fats that we might find in dairy or meat products can also make sebum thicker. A poor diet can cause an imbalance of these fat molecules and can decrease the quality of oil a single sebocyte can produce. This is the reason why having "oily skin" is not a precondition to having acne. The quality and viscosity of sebum are more important than the total produced quantity.

Indeed, some researchers have found no difference in total sebum production between acne patients and the general population [337], results which are the complete opposite to popular belief. Even if your skin secretes less sebum than on average, you are still at risk of developing acne if you have an imbalance in the ingredients that make up sebum.

At this point, it's important to mention that pore blockages are not necessarily harmful on their own; there's another ingredient that needs to be added to facilitate the formation of pimples. It's not bacteria, as you might guess, but pressure.

If a blockage does occur and gunky material gets trapped within our skin, this won't produce an inflamed pimple on its own. If left alone, these blockages will naturally clear themselves after some time and will only manifest themselves as tiny black dots on our skin (appropriately named *blackheads*). Their black color comes from the oxidation process that occurs when pore clogs come into contact with air. These obstructions are harmless and less visible than regular pimples, and simple facial scrubs can quickly clear them.

Although pore clogs are harmless on their own, if the pressure inside builds up enough, the outer skin layer will eventually rupture, spewing all the trapped gunk deeper within the skin.

Sebum production doesn't stop once a cap is formed. It will continue to be pumped until the pressure is so large that tiny skin ruptures will form. If this happens, the sebum (alongside any bacteria formed in the meantime) is free to enter deeper layers of our skin, activating the immune system and triggering inflammation. This process is summarized in Figure 17.

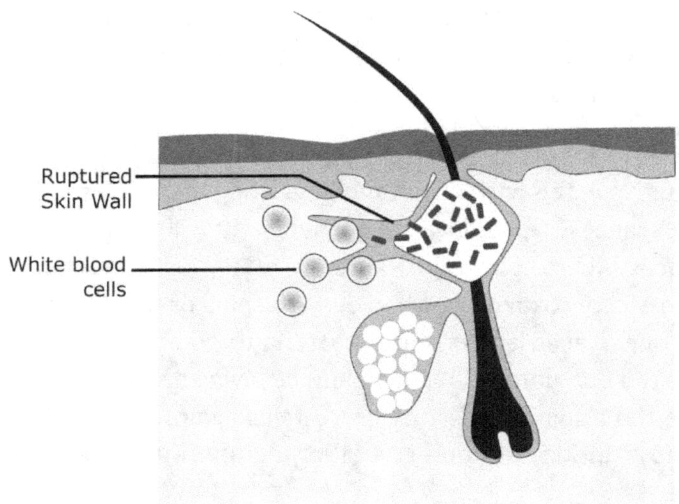

Figure 17 - Ruptured skin wall

Although sebum on its own will cause inflammation if infiltrated in our skin, when it's mixed with other foreign pathogens (such as bacteria), the effect will be much more pronounced [208].

A common bacterium thought to trigger this inflammatory response is *Cutibacterium acnes* (C. acnes). What sets this bacteria apart from most organisms in its class is that it can thrive in places devoid of oxygen, making blocked skin pores the perfect breeding ground.

Usually, C. acnes feeds on sebum to produce an acidic substance that can kill off other foreign pathogens. This secretion is mixed with the oily sebum, which helps plant it firmly on our skin, thus forming the first line of defense against microbes. In normal conditions, having C. acnes on our skin is actually beneficial. By eating sebum, C. acnes produces an acidic mantle that protects us against other, more harmful germs.

The problems come when C. acnes is left to over-multiply. Because C. acnes feeds on sebum, when a pore blockage occurs and bacteria get trapped within, it creates the perfect condition for C. acnes to overmultiply. If these colonies penetrate deep within our skin, it stimulates the release of pro-inflammatory signaling proteins, thus causing pimples.

Unintuitively, this problem is amplified when there is *less* oil on the skin. Because C. acnes loves to eat sebum, it will naturally migrate to places where it can get more of it. If you excessively scrub sebum off your skin – like when over-washing or when using soaps – the only places left for these bacteria to go and get sebum are within the skin pores [332]. Instead of thriving on our skin, helping create the acidic mantle that protects us against germs, C. acnes will move inside skin pores, multiplying and making acne much worse.

This is the reason why treating acne can be a frustrating experience for those who do not fully understand this disease. At first glance, it might seem like acne is a hygiene problem, one which could easily be solved by simply taking better care of our skin. In reality, hygiene is not as important as the factors that dictate how viscous the sebum is and how ramped up your immune system is at the site of the injury. Everything needed to form a pimple – the cap material, the bacteria, and the inflammation signaling proteins – is self-contained within these tiny hair chambers. If one tries to cure acne by excessively scrubbing their face (or using oil solvents, such as soap), they will only make the problem worse, as more bacteria migrate within skin pores worsening pimples once a skin rupture does occur.

This doesn't necessarily mean that hygiene doesn't play *some* role in acne formation, but just that it's not the most important factor. You will likely get the most bang for your buck by first targeting the intra-body processes that lead up to pimples rather than trying to clear acne using only lotions. The biggest improvement to your skin's health is made by using a combination of dietary changes and skin cleaning techniques.

Does washing your face help?

Even if acne is a disease driven primarily by internal bodily processes, some experiments have shown that regular face washing can improve acne slightly. Even so, not all techniques or products are equal. Which one is the best is still unclear, even though some swear by some brand or skincare product.

More than 1 in 5 women in the US use four or more facial skincare products in a typical day, with the most commonly used products being facial cleansers, lip products, and moisturizers [338]. It's no wonder that the entire skincare market is projected to be worth $183 billion by 2025 [339]. That is more than the GDP of some nations, including Hungary [340].

The fact that the skincare industry is worth so much is the primary reason why it's surprisingly hard to find unbiased research on specific cosmetic products. These studies are usually funded by the company which produces the product itself and, in some cases, even reviewed by these companies before publishing.

Take, for example, a study aimed at evaluating the efficacy against acne of a skincare routine that incorporates multiple products from the same brand (Golderma). The study was funded by the same company which manufactured these products, and, after the trial was completed, an "internal review by Galderma was completed to evaluate for accuracy of content prior to submission to the journal" [341]. I trust you see the irony in having the company which manufactures the product review and approve the results before publication.

Because most research in the skin-care industry is privately funded, there's not enough motivation from these companies to fund research for products that are not easily bottled or sold to regular consumers. Water, for example, hasn't been studied as of yet for its efficacy against acne. Obviously, this is because pharmaceutical companies have no incentive to perform research on something you can't put a label on (although the Bottled Water industry has done just this). If an experiment finds that water is just as effective at combating acne as pharmaceuticals, this will destroy entire companies or even industries.

Although water itself hasn't been tested so far, we do have some hints about the efficacy of generic face cleansers against acne. Through some recent experiments, we also have some suggestions regarding the optimal number of times we should wash our face.

We get these insights through a study that gave a group of acne sufferers a generic cleanser with no active ingredients to use for eight weeks as the only treatment for their acne. The participants were split further into three groups, in which the washing frequency varied from once to four times daily. All the patients were asked to wash twice daily in the first two weeks of the experiments, so they all had an equal start.

As shown in the figure below, the group with the biggest improvement was the one washing twice daily, while the one washing only once daily saw a slight worsening in total lesion count [332].

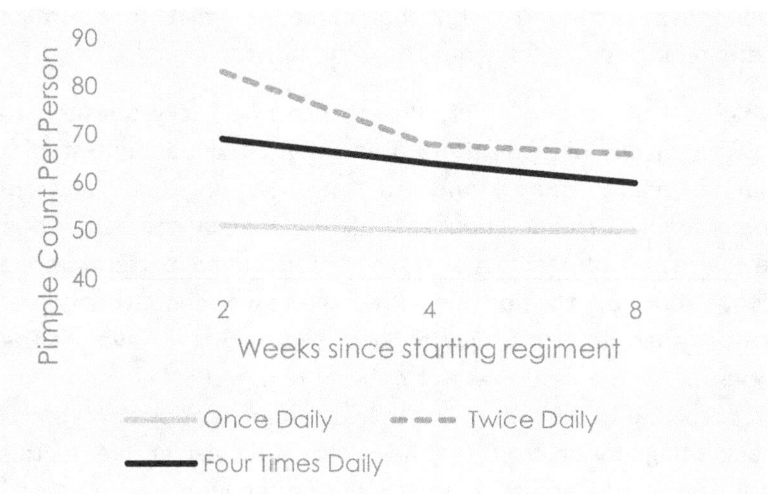

Figure 18 – Washing frequency effect on acne

It should be noted that this experiment tested a particular brand of face cleanser. Although it didn't contain any active ingredients, the fact that the researchers didn't try any other skincare product puts into question just how relevant these results are for other products. More so, the study was quite small, including only 34 male participants, meaning we shouldn't consider these results as definitive proof until more research is done on this topic.

After washing frequency, the next question you might have is which specific product is more effective at combating acne. After all, there are many brands of cleansers, face washes, soaps, and lotions, so it would be impossible for us to try them all until we find one that works.

The best group of products you can use are those that contain active ingredients. We've already mentioned the most important ones in this book, but benzoyl peroxide, tea tree oil, and mangosteen extract have been proven independently to improve acne in some way. They either kill the C. acnes bacteria itself, subvert your immune system not to be so sensitive to foreign pathogens, or change the quality of the sebum.

Which specific brand or product to use is a tricky question to answer, mainly because there aren't many independent studies that compare one brand to another. In the field of pharmaceuticals, experiments are usually done by companies that have a vested interest in making their product look better than the competition. Because of this, either the experiments themselves are designed in such a way to sway the results in favor of the sponsors, or the results aren't publicly released at all if they are not favorable to the brand. The only recommendation that we can make is to go for products that have known active ingredients. This includes generics as well, as they are just effective as name brands, as long as they contain the right proportions of active ingredients.

Picking and scaring

For most of us, acne is a short-lived disease, lasting on average for just two years [342]. Because it's short-lived, most people affected by this illness do not seek medical help, and if they do, they do so for a single session [343].

However, even if the disease itself heals in a relatively short time, the mental and physical scars can be long-lasting and, in some cases, permanent. We will discuss the psychological effects of this disease in the following few chapters, but the physical scars can serve as a permanent reminder of the distress imposed by this disease. These remnants can be so severe in some cases that they can cause more hardship than acne itself, leading to depression, low self-esteem, and social phobia [344]. Because of this, it is becoming increasingly apparent that, for patients diagnosed with acne, it's not enough just to treat the primary disease itself but also any secondary physical traumas resulting from the original pimples.

Scaring occurs when a wound cannot heal cleanly, either because the injury itself is too severe or because it's not left to heal correctly. For acne, scars usually form when pimples are not left alone and are continually picked open.

The number one priority of the human body is to close open wounds to prevent infections and complications. It will do so at any cost, even if it means leaving the injury permanently disfigured.

The process of wound healing is quite complex but can be broken down into three major stages. First, the site of injury is filled with blood, allowing reparation cells to inundate the affected area and start the healing process. Afterward, a thin protective bridge is formed, which connects the top-most layer of the skin and prevents germs and viruses from entering deeper within the body. After the first protective layer is formed, the wound can continue healing until completion.

The same process applies to pimple wounds as well. If a pimple is popped, this leaves a large hole in the skin, which needs to be healed quickly to prevent inflammation. Immediately after a pimple is popped, blood will flow to the affected area to fill it up with reparatory cells and to create the first protective bridge at the top of the injury. Clotting agents will start hardening the deposited blood, making a strong barrier against pathogens.

However, this barrier is still mostly temporary, as it's formed by hardened blood and not by final living skin cells. After around 12 hours from the initial trauma, the top-most layer of the skin will start to heal itself by creating a more permanent protective film using living skin cells. Only once this barrier is completed can the final wound healing process start. Afterward, structural and functional skin cells are made at the site of injury, rebuilding the skin layer, putting life back into the skin.

Although the healed tissue will never be as good as the original skin, if the wound is allowed to go through all healing stages normally and if the initial opening is not too large, the scar will not be noticeable to the naked eye. The problems start when the healing process is not allowed to run its usual course.

Sometimes, the wound is subjected to mechanical forces (such as picking at a pimple), whereby the top-most skin layer is damaged or never allowed to be created fully. In these cases, the protective bridge will not be flush with the rest of the skin, creating visible wells and scars.

If pimples are not allowed to heal correctly, either V-shaped (ice-pick), U-shaped (rolling), or box-shaped (boxcar) scars are formed. These will rarely heal on their own and will require expensive and invasive treatments, such as shooting lasers at the damaged area, sanding off the top-most layer of the skin, or chemically dissolving the scars with strong acids. These really don't sound like pleasant experiences, and it's best if we avoid these situations altogether.

At this point, it would be easy for me to say that the best way to avoid long-lasting scars is to stop picking at inflamed pimples. However, for some, this is not an easy feat to accomplish. Similar to how some people obsessively bite their nails or excessively wash their hands, some also compulsively pick at their pimples. This behavior is now even recognized as a neurological disorder, aptly named *skin picking disorder* (SPD), and often requires professional medical help to correct.

SPD is much more common in women than in men, with an estimated female-to-male ratio of around 8:1 [345]. Some data suggests that 16.6% of the population has excessively picked at their pimples at some point in their life, making it a much more common disease than what might seem at first glance [346].

Despite this disease being so widespread, the majority of those affected do not recognize it as a real affliction and do not seek medical help. Only around 5% of suspected chronic pickers are referred to a psychologist or psychiatrist [345]. Most dermatologists will acknowledge that picking is caused by the acne condition itself when, in reality, SPD is rooted much deeper than this. It has been suggested that SPD is caused by the intersection between acne and a primary psychiatric disorder, such as depression or obsessive-compulsive disorder.

The tendency to pick at a wound usually predates acne itself, and pimples are just an easy way to satisfy this need [347]. At the extreme end of this disease, some people will pick at pimples until severe scars are formed, even if they have minimal acne to begin with. This syndrome – called *acne excoriée des jeunes filles* – is common in young women with immature personalities.

If you have these symptoms or know someone who displays excessive picking, please take this condition seriously. SPD can lead to permanent disfigurement from acne scars that never heal on their own and are very difficult to treat. Even more, because SPD is an indication of another potentially more severe psychiatric disorder, people with SPD can have a decreased quality of life even after the primary acne condition is treated.

Depression and anxiety have been suggested to be the primary cause of SPD [348], and most patients are not aware of this trigger. It is also believed that excessive picking might be a protective device for some, as a coping mechanism for depressive episodes, or as a way to seek help for psychological distress. For these reasons, it's paramount to treat excessive picking on its own so that these factors that can decrease the quality of life of acne sufferers will not persist after acne is healed.

Mechanical Acne

Because acne is an inside-out disease (pimples form deep within the skin without the help of external forces), we have very few reasons to believe that touching or rubbing one's face will make this condition worse. However, this is true only up to a certain point. If you go out of your way and excessively rub your face (or any part of your body), you give rise to a particular form of acne, named *acne mechanica* [349], that has very little in common with the usual type of acne explored so far in this book.

As the name implies, acne mechanica is caused by excessive mechanical forces applied directly to the skin. This includes actions such as rubbing, heating, or extreme pressure. Acne mechanica isn't as studied as the standard form of this disease (mostly because it's much more easily treated), meaning we don't fully understand how and why it forms. However, because it's easily treatable, it's not that big of a concern for those that have it. More so, the pimples caused by excessive mechanical forces appear on places of the human body that are usually hidden, such as the buttocks or back, which is why most people simply ignore it and do not take active steps to treat this illness.

Acne mechanica has very little in common with regular acne, other than the fact that both diseases tend to happen to the same people [349]. If you have regular breakouts on your face, you are also at higher risk of developing acne mechanica as well, but on other regions of your body. It seems like this link is strongest in people who have highly inflamed pimples, pointing towards a predisposition towards inflammation as a common root cause for both diseases.

Acne mechanica looks very similar to regular acne, so it's easy to mistake one for the other. The only real difference between the two diseases is their root cause. Regular acne is caused by all the complex internal processes we've learned through this book, while acne mechanica is caused by excessive physical touching.

It's important to note that neither oily fingers nor dirt have anything to do with acne mechanica. Pimples of this type happen even if you rub your skin against clean and fresh clothes. Cleanliness and personal hygiene still aren't to blame for this form of acne either.

As for exact causes, there are many types of actions that can lead to excessive rubbing or heating of the skin. For example, extensively sitting on a chair will create constant pressure in just one spot. If you apply this pressure for long enough, then you can develop acne mechanica on your buttocks. Below, you can find a list of the most common actions and habits that can lead to acne mechanica, depending on the region where the breakout is happening [349]:

Face: supporting your head (with hands or through other means), rubbing with hands or fingers, athletic equipment (like chin straps, helmets, headbands), hats.

Neck: shirt collars and other clothing with neckbands (turtleneck), backpacks and straps, violins.

Shoulders: backpack straps, football pads.

Arms and Legs: orthopedic casts, rubbing and kneading of skin, rubbing inner thighs (especially common in individuals who are overweight)

Back and Chest: backrests of chairs (and seating in general), bras and bra straps, belts (especially wide ones), backpacks and straps, tight-fitting clothes.

Buttocks: chairs, seats, and general excessive sitting.

Diagnosing acne mechanica is not as obvious as you might think, as some of the actions that lead to this disease are unconscious, and it can take another person to point out that we have such a habit. However, once the trigger is known, treatment is pretty straightforward – simply eliminate the source of friction or heat. This can either be done by making a habit conscious, by not sitting in the same place for too long (also good for your general health), wearing loose-fitting clothes when walking, and so on.

Most people get mild forms of this illness and don't bother to treat it all. Because it's such a manageable disease to treat, researchers haven't made much effort in studying it either, hence why we don't know a lot about how it forms. As a result, most of the information we have on this disease dates back from the 1960s and 1970s, and it's unlikely we will get any new groundbreaking data anytime soon.

Either way, acne mechanica is a real disorder and, although it's rare to have blemishes caused by physical force on the face, it should be considered a potential root cause if you have acne. Some people are also at higher risk of developing acne mechanica, such as truck drivers, people who use the gym frequently, or office workers. If you find that your acne always happens in the same spot (on the shoulders or chin), or if it's seasonal (it only comes during sports season), you should check whether you have a habit of resting your chin on your hands for too long, or if your clothes are excessively tight.

As for regular acne, contrary to what is commonly thought, the actual causes of this disease have very little to do with cleanliness and personal hygiene. Even in extreme cases of touching and rubbing resulting in acne mechanica, the pimples are easily diagnosed and treated. If you do the minimum to keep your face reasonably clean (e.g., washing twice daily with a mild cleanser), then the forces that give rise to your pimples are very likely internal. Obsessively worrying about keeping strict cleansing routines will do more harm than good, especially if we ignore other aspects of this disease that are much more applicable and which have a more significant impact on our overall wellbeing.

CHAPTER SUMMARY

- Pimples form when thick sebum fails to flow freely out skin pores, creating blockages. The bacteria that gets trapped inside overmultiplies, causing inflammation if the outer skin layer is ruptured.

- Because acne forms within the skin, outside dirt or grease have minimal impact on this disease. There's no evidence to suggest that touching one's face can cause acne.

- One experiment found that washing the face twice daily with a mild cleanser can improve acne symptoms.

- Overwashing can be harmful, as more bacteria migrate within skin pores, where they can multiply freely.

- Picking pimples can cause long-term scars, which will not heal on their own. Excessive picking is usually a sign of an underlying psychiatric disorder, such as anxiety or depression, which should be treated separately.

- Severe rubbing or pressure on the skin can cause a different kind of acne, named acne mechanica. Although not well understood, acne mechanica is treated by simply removing the source of friction.

POLLUTION

As you read through this book, you might have felt that it's near impossible to escape acne. It seems that almost everything we eat can harm our skin. Dairy, meat, sugary foods, carbohydrates — virtually all major food groups are thought to interplay with acne in some way, making this disease almost unavoidable to those who follow a standard Western diet. Although the reality is not that grim, as there are only a couple of food groups that should be avoided, we still have to take one step further into this gloomy trend and say that the very act of breathing can be bad for our skin.

Most people are aware that air pollutants are harmful to our health. Even if we ignore the long-term climate risks these pollutants pose, air contaminants have become such an issue that 91% of the entire world's population lives in areas that exceed the recommended pollutants limits imposed by the World Health Organization. In 2019, it was estimated that around 4.2 million people die each year due to air pollution [350].

Contaminants in the air we breathe are linked with many adverse health effects, including lung cancer, strokes, and heart disease [350]. Although not well understood, the health implications of living in a polluted area are undeniable. And, because air pollution is associated with a wide range of diseases, it only makes sense to look at the implication to our skin as well.

The term "pollution" has come to mean many different things over the years, but it is generally defined as any contamination of the natural environment that we live in — be it the land, sea, or air. Humanity has been quite good at preventing land and sea pollution (except for fish, which are frequently contaminated with heavy metals [351]), but airborne particles are easily transmissible and are the most common pollution source we are exposed to. This includes substances that are directly harmful to our health and gasses that affect the general environment that we live in (e.g., greenhouse gasses).

Air pollutants are usually split into three major groups:

Gases - such as Ozone (O_3), Nitrogen Dioxide (NO_2), Carbon Dioxide (CO_2), Carbon Monoxide (CO), and Sulphur Dioxide (SO_2). These chemicals are gasses at room temperature, meaning they diffuse and spread easily through the air we breathe. All such gasses are toxic in high enough quantities, but usually, only Ozone, Nitrogen Dioxide, and Sulphur Dioxide are tracked for safety. They are not the most dangerous chemicals that we can be exposed to, but they are very common in industrialized nations. They are produced in abundance by certain human-made activities, such as by industrial processes or from vehicles.

Small airborne particles (often called Particulate Matter – PM) - are tiny particles of matter, be it organic or inorganic in origin, that are so small that they can quickly become airborne and travel for long distances in the air. Their exact source or chemical composition isn't as important as for gases, as the adverse effects are mechanical in nature. Particles that are between 2.5μm and 10μm in diameter (also called coarse particles, or PM10) are ten times smaller than the width of a human hair and can easily bypass the body's natural defenses against foreign objects. After dodging nose hairs and mucus, they enter our lungs, where they can cause inflammation and other damage [352]. As you can imagine, if enough such particles accumulate in our lungs, they can cause long-term adverse health effects that have been associated with a shortened life expectancy [353]. Particles that have a diameter smaller than 2.5μm (called fine particles, or PM2.5) are especially dangerous to our health, as they can also enter the bloodstream and, from there, travel anywhere in the body. These, too, have been shown to reduce life expectancy [353].

Volatile organic compounds (VOCs) - are substances that evaporate very quickly when exposed to the atmosphere. More than 10,000 chemicals are classified as VOCs, so it would be impossible to mention them all in this chapter. However, they are usually produced when using solvents or chemicals at home or in offices – think of the smell you get when spray painting. Common health effects include irritation of the eyes, nose, and throat, but it can lead to even worse side effects.

Pollution doesn't affect all countries of the world equally. Compared to 30 years ago, most Western nations have taken active steps to reduce airborne pollutants to the point where the health costs are negligible. However, nations that are still in development have put more emphasis on improving economic conditions to the detriment of citizens' health. Particularly, the most affected countries by air pollution are those that are currently experiencing rapid economic growth and which are situated in Southeast Asia, Africa, and India. This is also the reason why most of the research linking air pollution to health deterioration has come from these countries.

There is even a website that shows how many years you would gain if you were to breathe non-polluted air, broken down by country. In places such as China and India, you would lose more than six years of your life just by living in the most polluted areas. You can visit the website here: https://tinyurl.com/pol-index

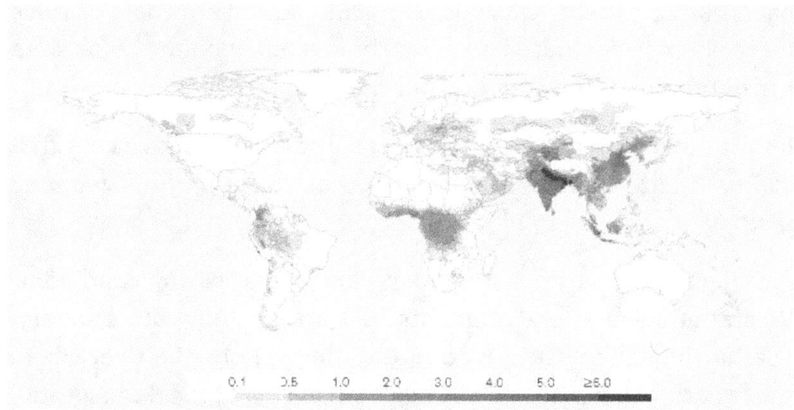

Figure 19 - Years lost due to air polution

(source: https://aqli.epic.uchicago.edu/the-index/)

Medical research in this area has provided overwhelming evidence that constant exposure to airborne pollutants can deteriorate our health [354]. Although the human body has evolved several defenses against environmental damage, these prove insufficient given the number of stressors modern society is producing. As it happens, most of our protection against pollution comes from our skin. Pollutants don't only bypass these defenses, but they also repress them, making us more prone to other diseases that would normally be blocked by these guards.

Humans have three primary defense mechanisms against environmental damage.

Foremost, there's the skin itself, which provides a physical barrier that protects us against mechanical or chemical damage. Our skin's outmost layer is made entirely of dead skin cells, helping us sustain physical damage without much harm to the rest of the organs. These dead skin cells can easily tear off without causing us pain.

On top of that, there's a thin layer of an oily mixture of acidic and antimicrobial substances that provides a chemical barrier against bacteria and other pathogens. The acidic ingredients help dissolve the cells of living invaders, while the oily component helps keep the entire mixture planted on our skin.

If these two barriers fail, humans can also deploy active cells that can neutralize threats, such as cells that are part of our immune system.

Although these barriers are enough for ordinary living conditions, Westerners live in environments that are anything but ordinary. The harmful chemicals found in the atmosphere can overwhelm these natural defenses, to the point of causing organ damage and, in some cases, death.

Some air-born pollutants are more harmful than others. Although small particulate matter can get lodged in our lungs and cause serious health problems (including cancer), they're relatively harmless to our skin [355]. The real danger for acne comes from certain gasses that are extremely reactive and which can cause excessive oxidative stress and cell damage. The most notorious of them all is ozone, an unstable oxygen molecule that is highly volatile and which is very often found in dense and polluted cities.

Most people have heard of ozone from the thin layer of this gas that sits at the top of our atmosphere, protecting us from harmful UV radiation. It became famous once it started to wither away from the overuse of certain human-made chemicals – such as refrigerants and various solvents – that interact with ozone to change its chemical composition. The famous ozone crisis from the 1970s is now mostly on track to being resolved, as ozone can continuously regenerate itself each year. After we became aware of the environmental damage refrigerants pose, we started being more conservative to their usage, allowing the ozone layer to heal itself. It is estimated that the ozone layer will recover entirely sometime in the 2030s [356].

Although ozone is protective when concentrated at the top of our atmosphere, it becomes harmful to our health if we come into contact with it and breathe it directly. Unfortunately for us, some modern industrial processes release alarmingly large quantities of ozone, which remain in the lower atmosphere, forcing humans to inhale this harmful chemical past safe levels.

Typically, ozone forms when highly energetic light particles hit a single oxygen atom, splitting it into two. Once in this state, oxygen is very unstable, and it seeks to join with other oxygen molecules to form a stable three-atom particle.

Before humans came along, this process of converting oxygen into ozone occurred primarily at the top of the atmosphere, when UV rays from the sun smash into oxygen molecules, breaking them apart. Because ozone is rarely found in nature, living creatures have evolved few defenses against this chemical.

With the advent of industrialization, finding clusters of ozone at lower levels of the atmosphere is much more common, especially in dense cities, and is extremely damaging to our health. In modern times, ozone is mainly formed as a byproduct of burning fossil fuels, particularly by internal combustion engines, putting more pockets of this harmful gas much closer to humans [357].

Ozone is much less stable than oxygen and is a powerful oxidant. It is so powerful that it has strong antibacterial properties, being used in some industries to kill bacteria and disinfect surfaces [358]. It can even corrode metal, which is why it's a problem for plumbing systems that use copper pipes [359]. As you can imagine, our soft tissue is no match for the metal corrosive powers of ozone. When it comes into contact with our skin, ozone can harm and bypass all three major defenses that we have against environmental damage.

On the one hand, ozone induces chemical changes to the outer oily layer that sits on our skin. These changes ultimately produce a mixture that can irritate and do damage to surrounding cells. When ozone comes into contact with sebum, it oxidizes certain constituents, thus making the entire blend more prone to blockages and more likely to induce acne. Particularly, ozone alters the chemical composition of squalene to produce oxides of this substance, which have been found to encourage inflammation, promote pore blockages, and increase the rate at which skin cells are created and die [360] [208]. All of this can exacerbate acne and make us more likely to break out.

Besides the interaction with squalene, ozone also affects our skin directly, further exacerbating acne. Although other gasses have oxidative abilities, what makes ozone especially dangerous is that it can infiltrate deeper within the skin, bypassing the initial layer of dead skin cells [361]. Once ozone penetrates this layer, it can induce several acne-promoting effects, including pro-inflammatory responses from our immune system and oxidative damage to skin cells [362].

As you can imagine, the human body will try to neutralize these highly reactive chemicals before they damage any internal tissue. This typically happens through the anti-oxidation process discussed in the

Fruits and Berries chapter, whereby neutralizing chemicals are released to join with these reactive molecules, thus defusing them. However, our defenses have limits; there are only so many anti-oxidants to go around. If our bodies can't keep up with the amount of oxidative damage these gases produce, we will eventually succumb to these harmful invaders. Once this happens, diseases that are generally prevented by anti-oxidants will start to develop.

In most cases, skin cells store enough anti-oxidants to deal with normal levels of reactive oxygen molecules that are created through the usual cellular processes. But, if enough external oxidants bombard our skin, this overwhelms our protective system, preventing its normal function.

In this state, the skin simply cannot keep up with the amount of damage these oxidants do, leading to inflammation and other acne-promoting effects [363]. Interestingly, one study found that a high dose of Vitamin C (a potent anti-oxidant) can prevent most of these harmful effects by decreasing oxidation levels by up to 90% [363]. This might mean that, if you simply can't avoid living in highly polluted areas, one way to prevent oxidative damage to the skin is to regularly consume products rich in Vitamin C (or antioxidants in general), such as fruits and legumes.

Ozone is not the only airborne pollutant thought to trigger acne. Recent evidence suggests that nitrogen dioxide can be equally harmful.

In one experiment, a group of researchers compared local air pollution levels with the rate at which pimples form in 64 participants. At the end of the 8-week study period, the researchers found that there was a *significant* connection between pollution levels and the rate at which sebum is produced. Interestingly, this effect was not instant. The research found that there was a one-week delay between when air pollutant levels peak and when subsequent pimples are formed [364]. The study didn't detail what might cause this acne aggravation, so the exact explanation for this effect is unknown. However, the link between acne and pollution was strongest with three different air contaminants, including PM2.5, PM10, and nitrous oxide.

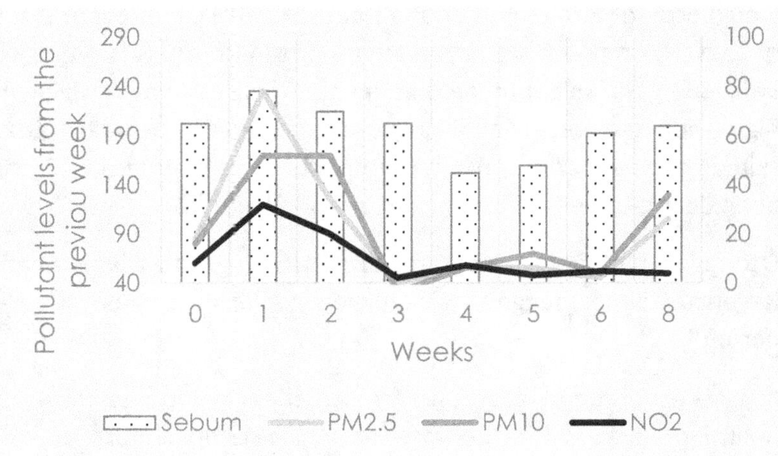

Figure 20 - Air pollutants effect on Sebum Levels

Another experiment, based in China, found that women who live in more polluted areas of the country had oilier skin than normal, which the researchers considered a risk factor for acne. The scientists analyzed the sebum secretion rate of women located in 5 different regions of the country. These regions had varying levels of air pollution levels and included the most polluted metropolis of all, namely Beijing. After analyzing the data, the scientists found that women who lived in more polluted areas had twice the sebum secretion rate compared to the other regions [365].

This is not necessarily proof that air pollution causes acne, but it at least provides a hint that something in the environment was causing the skin of these women to be more stressed. More so, regions that are more polluted also tend to be richer than average, as air pollution is usually a sign of higher industrialization and economic activity. This means that the women who lived in more polluted cities likely also had higher living conditions, meaning they were able to afford more acne-inducing foods, such as sweets, meats, or dairy.

Despite the limitations in these experiments, the idea that exposure to pollution leads to acne is quite widespread among professionals in the healthcare space. A survey among dermatologists in Beijing found that 67% of respondents believed that acne worsens during days with more air pollution [362]. This belief does stem from really, as some investigations using data on hospital visits have shown that dermatologic clinics see an influx of acne patients on highly polluted days.

In one such analysis, a group of researchers looked at the number of visits to certain dermatology clinics, which were compared to the air pollution levels several days before the hospital visit. This experiment was based in Beijing, one of the most polluted regions on Earth. The researchers looked at several indicators of air pollution, including particulate matter (PM25 and PMM10), nitrogen dioxide (NO_2), and sulfur dioxide (SO_2). The study was performed on data recorded between 2012 and 2014 and included almost 60,000 patient visits.

After they tallied up the numbers, the researchers did, in fact, find a significant correlation between visits to dermatologists and air pollutants. Notably, the strongest association was found with NO_2, while SO_2 was actually found to be protective. On days in which NO_2 concentrations were higher, more hospital visits were recorded. Inversely, on days in which SO_2 levels were higher, *fewer* clinic visits were recorded. This effect was strongest 1-2 weeks after pollution levels peaked, indicating, once more, that these pollutants take some time before they reach their highest irritating abilities and that there is a slight delay between exposure to contaminants and acne breakout [366].

It should be noted that the effect is not major. A doubling of NO_2 levels only increased patient visits by 2.5%. This tiny increase in acne risk pales in comparison to the other risk factors we've looked at so far in this book – and this is for a region far more polluted than typical Western cities. How worried you should be about air pollution in regards to acne is unclear. Although we know that certain chemicals irritate the skin when tested in isolated environments, it's still unknown just how severe this effect is when we are exposed to real-world air pollution, especially for regions that sit below the recommended levels published by the WHO.

Even though the link between pollution and acne is still unclear, the overall health implications of constant exposure to air contaminants are undeniable. Small particulate matter has been found to increase the risk of developing cardiovascular and respiratory diseases (such as asthma, chronic bronchitis, rhinitis, lung development), neurological debilitation, diabetes, atherosclerosis, and others [367]. The effect is so dramatic that, in the most polluted cities, inhabitants who are chronically exposed to elevated air pollution levels have a shortened life by up to 6 years.

There is strong evidence that air pollution is one of the main contributing factors for early death in modern times. Although acne is on the list of probable harmful effects from exposure to air pollution, other health implications are more pronounced and more damaging, signaling a need to drive down this human-made killer even further. Progress has been made in certain parts of the world, particularly in Western Europe and North America, but other regions of the globe are not taking this threat seriously. They are continuing to pump pollutants at an ever-increasing rate, effectively killing their citizens. Although there is very little we can do as individuals to protect ourselves against this invisible killer, we can all invest in our long-term health by supporting measures and lifestyle changes that help drive down air contamination.

CHAPTER SUMMARY

- Air pollution is a combination of many different kinds of harmful gasses and airborne particles. Of these, ozone and nitrogen dioxide have been linked with acne

- Ozone is especially harmful, as it can alter the chemical composition of sebum to make it more prone to pore blockages while also promoting inflammation. Ozone is also a potent source of oxidative stress, further irritating the skin.

- High dosages of antioxidants (such as Vitamin C) can protect us against oxidative damage caused by air pollution.

- There is some evidence that suggests that people living in highly polluted areas are more likely to develop acne. However, this effect is only marginal and unlikely to be the main cause of acne.

STRESS

If you're reading this book, chances are you are suffering from acne. If this is true, I don't have to tell you just how much mental strain this disease can create, and that the repercussions of having pimples are more than just "skin deep." Because this disease affects such a large percentage of the population (usually during critical times of personal development), this has meant that the phycological and social tolls this disease brings upon its sufferers can, in many cases, outweigh the adverse effects brought on by the disease itself.

Acne is still poorly understood, even among medical professionals. One study found that 25% of medical students believed that poor hygiene was the leading cause of acne [368], even though we now know this to be false. Considering that this study was performed on people who have much more medical knowledge than the average person, it's clear that these misconceptions are still widespread. The fact that so many people believe this disease is caused by "being dirty" and "not washing enough" can create social stigmas against those who are vulnerable.

It also doesn't help that the areas of the skin that are more prone to breaking out are critical to social interactions and really the first thing we notice when we meet someone new. Acne wouldn't be the global problem it is today, and the pharmaceutical industry for this disease wouldn't be worth 20 billion USD [4] if pimples formed in areas that are easier to conceal, such as the back or stomach. When we also consider that acne is more common during adolescence – a critical time for socializing and personality development – it's easy to see why acne can give rise to long-lasting scars, both physically and mentally.

All of these factors — misconceptions about what causes acne, uneven distribution on the body, social stigma, development during early adolescence, Western culture obsession with physical appearances, frustration with treatments that don't work — they conspire to induce severe mental health problems in those affected, including symptoms of depression, anxiety, and generally lower quality of life. These side effects are not rare. In fact, they are quite common [369]. People with acne are two to three times more likely to have clinical depression compared to the general population [369].

The negative implications of acne do not stop at just mental health issues but can also creep up in many different places of our lives. Be it because we are subconsciously biased against people with acne marks, or maybe because acne makes people less confident, it was found that those with acne are more likely to be unemployed. Sufferers of acne have 65% to 76% higher unemployment rates compared to normal [370]. Although the reason for this is unclear, the implications are undeniable. Acne has far wider repercussions than what is evident, both for the individual and for society as a whole.

Preventing these negative influences on our mental wellbeing is a complex problem to tackle, mainly because the link between acne and mental health is not a simple straight arrow. One can see why acne can cause depression and anxiety but is the reverse also true? Does the stress induced by acne conspire to aggravate this disease even more, thus creating a self-feeding snowball? To answer these questions, we must look at both parts of the equation separately.

Acne causes stress

In 2001, 215 final-year medical students were asked to write a short essay, starting from the following fictional story:

An 18-year-old female who works as a model comes to see you with moderately severe papulopustular acne. She has a marked premenstrual flare of her acne.

a. What factors may have exacerbated her acne?

b. Describe the treatment options available for her acne.

Take a moment to think about what you would answer if you were one of the 215 medical students. Even though we still have some topics to cover in this book, base your answer only on the acne risk factors presented so far.

How well do you think you stack up against professional medical practitioners?

In the end, 79% of respondents thought that hormones caused by changes in the menstrual cycle had something to do with the acne breakout. This is expected, as the model presented in the fictive example linked their acne flare-up with her premenstrual cycle, which is known to alter normal hormonal levels [368]. Don't worry if this wasn't your first guess – we will cover hormones as a potential acne trigger in the final chapter of this book.

The second most popular answer was stress, mentioned by 67% of the students. The third most cited cause was topical sources (like makeup or poor facial hygiene), brought up by 59% of respondents. Dietary factors came in fourth, mentioned by 41% of students. Hopefully, by this time, you've gained a different perspective on this disease and have put this last item higher up on your list.

Given the widespread myth that cleanliness is a significant cause of acne, it shouldn't be surprising that the most common suggested treatment given by the medical students was hygiene-related. The top recommended non-pharmaceutical treatment was improved facial care, mentioned by 78% of respondents. This included recommendations to apply cleansers more often and to reduce cosmetic usage. Improving the diet wasn't mentioned by any of the respondents.

This myth that being dirty causes pimples is a double edge sword. On the one hand, being mislead about acne triggers and potential remedies will mean you will devote your money and energy *on the wrong* treatment. Believing that washing your face will cure your condition, sticking to a thorough and often expensive skincare routine, and then not seeing results will drive anyone crazy.

What's more, even if you do understand the mechanisms of acne, that doesn't mean others will as well. This can cause you to be inundated with unhelpful suggestions, such as "change your pillowcase daily" or "stop touching your face." Although well-intentioned, being constantly bombarded by unhelpful advice from friends and family can lead to a constant state of frustration. Most who are not affected by acne will not devote the same energy to understanding this disease as someone whose life is impacted by this illness. For this reason, acne sufferers will likely continue to be perceived as "dirty" and "greasy" for the foreseeable future, which puts a significant dent in the self-confidence of those affected.

All of these myths and misconceptions have made psychological distress an incredibly common side effect among people with acne. One study found that 44% of acne patients had *clinically* significant anxiety, while 18% were depressed. Both anxiety and depression are much more common among acne sufferers compared to the general population. Acne even beats most other skin conditions, including psoriasis, on the number of psychological side effects [2]. What's more, the severity of these mental health issues is directly correlated with the severity of acne. The worse the breakout is, the more likely it is for one to be depressed.

To quantify precisely how depressed or anxious one is, a system called the *Hospital Anxiety and Depression Scale* (HADS) is used among medical practitioners. This score is calculated by asking patients to fill out a simple questionnaire that measures how likely one is to perform actions that are strongly associated with depression or anxiety, such as watching a lot of TV or not caring too much about one's appearance. A value between 8 and 10 is considered "borderline abnormal," while anything over 11 is regarded as clinical depression or anxiety. You can easily find online surveys if you're curious about your own HADS score.

To find out if there is a link between acne severity and how depressed one is, one group of Chinese researchers asked 2,000 high school pupils to fill out a questionnaire that can determine their HADS score. This score was then compared with the pupils' acne history. Because acne is widespread among young adults and adolescents, the scientists had a good ratio of students suffering from acne and students with clear skin.

When the researchers compared the scores between the two groups, they were able to find that depressive tendencies correlate with the severity of acne. Clear-skin pupils had an average HADS score of 3.85 (well below the limit for depression), while students with a more severe form of acne had an average score of 8.12 (borderline depression) [371].

What's more, depressive tendencies increased linearly with the severity of acne. The more pimples the students had, the worse the depression was. Those who had only light forms of acne had a HADS score below 7, while those with severe acne had a depression score of over 8.

The same trend was found for anxiety as well. Students with acne were more anxious than average, and these negative feelings increased as acne worsened. Considering that similar results were found in other studies performed in Iraq [372], Turkey [373], and France [374], there's an undeniable link between acne and psychological distress.

Feelings of being ugly or disfigured will make anyone more recluse. This can have ramifications in people's lives and society as a whole by making acne sufferers less likely to engage in activities or hobbies that involve social interactions. Students with acne were found to skip school more often and tended to avoid hobbies that required taking one's clothes off (like swimming). One study found that 13% of acne patients reported a decline in school performance caused by their condition, 30% had marriage issues, while 17% said they had trouble finding friends [375]. A similar study from China found that students with acne were more likely to be victims of peer bullying, be involved in an intra-family conflict, suffer from academic stress or failure, and be discriminated against [371].

Depression and anxiety caused by acne is not just "in your head" and can't be treated easily without professional help. These feelings can be amplified by the behavior of others, either from discrimination or from active bullying. It has real ramifications in people's lives, leading to academic or economic failure, affecting not only the individual but also society as a whole.

These implications will only get worse as Western civilizations become more obsessed with beauty and physical perfection. When was the last time you saw a magazine put someone with acne on their covers? For these reasons, suicide rates are significantly higher in people with acne than in the general population. One study reported that acne patients were twice as likely to have suicidal thoughts compared to normal [376].

Why can acne be bad for your mental health	Possible complications
• Distributed mostly on the face • Social stigma around appearance • Usually first appears in adolescence • Widespread misconceptions around what causes acne	• Clinical depression and anxiety • Low self-esteem • Impaired social life • Generally reduced quality of life • Higher suicide rates

The good news is that these mental health issues will largely go away if acne is treated. One research found that anxiety and depression scores do improve once patients are cured of their primary disease. The group of researchers measured anxiety scores of acne sufferers before and after starting treatment. Before medication, the patients had an average anxiety score of 9, while a quarter of respondents had a score of over 11, which is considered clinically severe. After treating acne, only about 3.5% of patients reported anxiety scores higher than 11 [375].

Although anxiety rates were not completely zero, the improvement to the quality of life of these acne patients was substantial. For this reason, it's essential to recognize these secondary mental health issues before they cause long-term harm to those affected and treat them early. Certain medical professionals now recommend using psychotherapy while treating acne to help prevent lingering depression or anxiety [377].

Although it has been found that treating acne will improve the mental wellbeing of those affected, for some people, actively taking acne medication can worsen their depression. There is a common myth that certain acne drugs can exacerbate feelings of depression or anxiety. Particularly, these myths revolve around the isotretinoin drug – one of the most common medications administered to acne patients.

It's hard to pinpoint the origins of this myth, but one potential source is the case of Charles Bishop, a 15-year-old who ultimately committed suicide while on this medication [378]. His death was quite violent and made headlines in several newspapers across the globe at that time. Weeks after 9/11, Charles purposely crashed his plane into a 42-story tall building, killing himself instantly. He had no prior history of depression or suicidal thoughts. The only explanation the family could find for his tragic demise was a recent switch to the isotretinoin drug to treat his acne condition. Charles' family was quoted saying: "This was psychotic and the only conclusion we have been able to draw is the Accutane poisoned him." This case has since been dismissed, but the evidence against isotretinoin has been piling up since then.

A recent review made on reports from the US Food and Drug Administration found 17,829 psychiatric adverse effects caused by isotretinoin, placing this drug as the fifth most common medication reported to the US Adverse Event Reporting System in relation to depression. Of these 17,000 cases, 42% were incidents of depression, 16% of emotional liability, and 13% of increased anxiety. More worryingly, the study also found that around 12% of these reports involved suicidal thoughts, while 3.3% were attempted suicides. Of the 17,000 reported cases of adverse health effects due to isotretinoin, 2.1% ended in suicide [379]. Sadly, the report showed that teenagers were much more likely to be affected by the drug. Almost half of all reported suicides were by adolescents.

These results were mirrored by a slightly older review of reported health issues due to isotretinoin. The study found symptoms of depressions improve once acne patients stop taking this drug, only to come back once they restart treatment [380]. However, this is mostly anecdotal evidence and isn't considered exactly proof.

More so, this research analyzed data spanning 20 years, so there's bound to be *some* suicides in such a large timespan. As you can imagine, a lot of people used acne treatments in this period, and some of them were naturally more depressed than others. If you calculate the suicide rate reported for all people taking isotretinoin during this time, it actually comes lower than the national average [381].

Although we don't have definitive proof that isotretinoin causes depression, we do have some in-vitro tests that give plausible explanations for why we see these effects.

One study found that retinoids (the class of drugs that isotretinoin is part of) can interfere with the dopamine system of the brain, which is generally considered the "feel good" region [382]. Dopamine is a hormone that is released when we accomplish certain tasks, giving us a feeling of achievement, thus motivating us to perform more similar rewarding tasks. If isotretinoin blocks the function of this hormone in the brain, it can lead to decreased motivation and a general lower sense of well-being, causing depression.

Similarly, in an experiment performed on mice, isotretinoin was found to significantly suppress cell division in the hippocampus, an area of the brain associated with learning and memory [383]. To test how well the mice in the experiment learn, they were put into the usual maze that they had to navigate to get a food reward. When put under these kinds of tests, mice usually learn the structure of the labyrinth after some time, making fewer and fewer errors as they traverse it. However, the mice that were given isotretinoin had a much harder time learning the layout of the maze, making twice as many errors as the control group. What's more, after performing biopsies on the brain, the researchers found that the brain of mice fed isotretinoin had 42% decreased regenerative activity of neurons.

Another study found that depression-like behaviors increase in mice that were administered isotretinoin. The researchers found a significant disruption in the serotonin hormone – a neurotransmitter involved in feelings of well-being and happiness [384]. Lastly, another experiment, but this time performed on adult humans, found that isotretinoin usage was associated with decreased brain metabolism in the orbitofrontal cortex, an area of the brain known to mediate symptoms of depression [385].

As you can see, there are many plausible explanations for why isotretinoin might cause depressive symptoms, putting into question the drug's safety in humans. The well-known Accutanate drug (which uses isotretinoin as the active ingredient) has been retracted due to health safety concerns, but other medicines that contain isotretinoin are still sold throughout the world.

This drug is very effective at treating acne, so it will likely continue being sold for the foreseeable future. The secondary health costs of continuing to use this drug are still being evaluated. Even so, anyone thinking of taking this medication should be well aware of the potential side effects to mood and learning so that they can consider other safer treatment options. One can argue that any medicine is a balance between the positive health effects they bring and the potential adverse side effects. Although this is true, isotretinoin is not the only option for treating acne, and it's easy to give in to desperation when you only want to get rid of pimples and don't care about the costs.

Even if we sideline isotretinoin for now, the link between acne and depression is undeniable. People suffering from this disease have higher depression and anxiety scores than average, are more likely to be unemployed, anc generally have a decreased quality of life. Therefore, dermatologists should take special care to recognize these secondary health implications and suggest appropriate treatment options before they create long-lasting mental scars.

We've seen that acne can cause depression and anxiety, but is the reverse also true? Can feelings of anxiety and stress cause acne, and, if true, can we improve acne by providing better coping mechanisms for the mental strain induced by this disease? We will find out in the next section.

Stress causes acne

We've previously seen that stress is a top choice among medical practitioners as a cause of acne. It seems that this idea that nervousness leads to a pimple is also quite common among the general population. One survey in Korea found that 82% of people with acne believed that stress and feelings of anxiety worsened their condition. This was their top choice, followed by lack of sleep and hormonal changes caused by menstruation [307]. Although this idea that stress causes people to breakout is quite common, proving it has shown to be quite tricky.

The link between stress and acne is undeniable, being recognized through numerous studies that find that people with acne also tend to be more stressed [200] [386] [172]. This makes sense when we put the previous section into perspective. People with acne are more self-conscious, are more prone to academic and career failure, and can develop compulsive behaviors, such as stress picking. Even clear-skin people experiencing these events would start to feel worried and anxious about their future.

Although this association is well established, the reverse is trickier to prove. To figure out if stress causes breakouts, one would need to purposefully take a group of people and put them under considerable mental strain to see if these feelings affect their skin's health. Because stressing people out for long periods can be considered "cruel," nobody has attempted this type of experiment until now.

Still, even if we can't make people feel more stressed, that doesn't mean we can't observe what happens through everyday life events. Some days are naturally more stressful than others, and we can use this to our advantage. Exams, public speaking, taking your driver's license, publishing your first book – are all events that are bound to make people feel more nervous. If stress does cause acne, we can follow people through these difficult life events and observe any difference in pimple counts that happen after going through these experiences. This is exactly what one group of British researchers investigated.

The researchers recruited a small sample of people, which were tracked throughout their normal lives, for a total of three months. During this experiment, stressful life events were recorded, alongside any acne flaring which might have occurred afterward. Although the sample size was too small to definitively prove that stress causes acne, the researchers did find that people who go through more "negative life events" had a higher frequency of acne cases [387].

Those who had pimples went through 40% more negative life events during the examination period. It should be noted that the researchers found no difference between people with and without acne regarding *total* stressful events, but only with circumstances that were deemed *undesirable*. Stressful events can also have a positive impact on one's life, such as getting married or having your first child. It seems like these beneficial events were not associated with an increased risk of developing acne.

Similar results were found by another study performed in Singapore, in which one group of researchers recruited students aged 15, which were then monitored for stressful life events and any subsequent acne breakouts. Normally, a student's life is a particularly stressful one, filled with exams, teasing, and bodily changes, making this group of people the ideal candidates for such an experiment. But these were no ordinary students. They were *Singaporean* students. The educational system in this country is renowned for producing some of the best graduates in the world, but for also being one of the most stressful systems you can participate in. So much so that there have been academic studies showing that stress levels significantly increase in students during examination periods in Singapore [388], which can take a severe toll on the health of the students.

Tragically, studies have also shown that youth suicide rates spike in Singapore during June and October, corresponding to academic terms in this country [389]. It is heartbreaking that young children are subjected to such psychological trials, even if this comes with higher school performance than average. Even so, the good news is that the educational system in Singapore has made recent changes to make exams more manageable, to hopefully improve the wellbeing of students from this country.

Unsurprisingly, the research performed on Singaporean students found that the pupils felt significantly more stressed during examination times. Interestingly, the stress levels were substantially higher for young boys than girls; the explanation for this could be that girls were more prepared for the exams. Although the researchers did not find a link between sebum levels and stress, they did note that acne severity increases during these stressful events [390]. During the examination period, the students had more pimples and of worse severity. This was true for both boys and girls, even if the girls reported lower stress levels overall.

The fact that sebum levels do not increase during stressful times is also a valuable clue as to what might cause anxiety-induced breakouts. If the bodily change that causes pimples is not sebum-related, then there might be some other internal processes that damage our skin, potentially exacerbating acne. We will come back to this idea later in this chapter.

This link between acne and stress is found not only when we look at short-term stressful life events but also in people who are regularly exposed to stress. For example, one study found that women who have stressful jobs also tend to have more acne. The study found that 59% of adult women with acne had challenging careers, twice as high as the general population [391]. The women with acne also reported significantly higher stress levels than the general population; 85% of women with acne reported moderate to severe stress levels.

All the evidence so far suggests that people who are generally more stressed also tend to flare up more often. If we put the previous section into perspective, which found that acne is a source of anxiety and stress, it's easy to see how this entire device can be considered a self-feeding machine, which, once started, is difficult to stop. If stress causes acne, and acne causes stress, how do we break this loop to improve both our physical appearance and our mental sanity?

To understand why feelings of stress can give way to acne breakouts, we must first understand how stress manifests itself in the human body. More importantly, we also need to check how the stress signal from our brain reaches our skin cells and why this can give rise to the dreaded pimples.

*

Most of us have heard of the "fight-or-flight" response, which is felt during dangerous situations. These feelings of acute stress can be beneficial at times, particularly in circumstances that might cost us our life. However, in modern times, these feelings of panic very rarely come when we are truly in danger. They are unhelpful more often than not.

The benefits we could get from feeling anxious have withered away since the early days of hunter-gathers. We no longer have to fight with wild animals to procure our food, and we no longer have to worry too much about finding a safe place to sleep. The unwanted reaction our skin has to stressful feelings is likely not intended and is just a byproduct of how the fight-or-flight signal gets transmitted throughout our body.

As you might have noticed, certain physiological changes occur within our bodies when we go through bouts of stressful events. Heart rate gets faster, we sweat more than usual, and our legs start to twitch. Other invisible internal changes occur as well, like a heightened immune system and increased glucose production.

When we feel stressed, the human body transforms existing deposits of fats and proteins into simpler sugars, increasing the reserves of glucose in our muscles to be used as energy in case of intense physical activities. All these changes prepare us to deal with potential dangers by giving us the energy we need to run from or towards wild animals. Similarly, if we are injured during challenging situations, the stress response also heightens our immune system to help us deal with any harm that might occur.

It's not by accident that we have evolved this way. Our ancestors that were more prepared to hunt for food or run away from danger had a better chance of surviving and passing down their genes. If there's an actual imminent threat we have to deal with, these bodily changes help us deal with dangerous situations better and are highly beneficial. But, if there's no real life-or-death threat, then chronic exposure to stress will do more harm than good in the long run. Prolonged feelings of anxiety have been shown to have long-lasting adverse health effects, including cognitive and memory decline, suppressed immune systems, insulin resistance [392], and even alcoholism [393].

These adverse health effects (including the potential ones to our skin) stem from the fact that the triggers that prepare us to go through dangerous situations should only be used as an emergency lever and not something we should be exposed to constantly.

This situation is similar to how car racing enthusiasts will increase the power of a car's engine by mixing the fuel and air that normally go into these engines with highly reactive gasses. This increases the mixture's burn rate, making the explosions that happen in engine cylinders much more powerful, thus increasing engine output and making the car go faster. Although this increases engine power for short periods, if the reactive gases are injected for too long, then the entire engine will blow up. The same analogy carries over to the human body when we are exposed to feelings of stress for too long. The heightened immune system will eventually start to attack healthy cells, leading to inflammation and chronic health problems as a result.

The same damaging effects carry over to our skin as well. The stress signal that prepares us to deal with imminent danger also triggers specific changes in the skin that make it more prone to breaking out.

This signal starts in the brain, which ultimately decides if we should feel anxious or not based on our environment. But this signal needs a way to travel to all organs the brain wants to affect, to increase the pulse rate, blood oxygen levels, and to put the immune system into overdrive. Part of this signal is transmitted through nerves, which are very precise and modify the behavior of just a single organ. But part of the message is also transmitted through imprecise hormones, which produces unintended changes in the organs that come into contact with these stress signals.

This information pipeline begins in the brain, in a region called the *hypothalamus.* This almond-size area is primarily responsible for linking the nervous system to the rest of the body by way of the *endocrine system* (a collection of hormones and hormone-sensing organs).

The hypothalamus contains multiple areas that can release hormones, each one with a unique role in normal bodily function. For example, oxytocin is released by the hypothalamus when we are aroused, vasopressin is released when we are feeling thirsty, and the *corticotropin-releasing hormone (CRH)* is produced when we are feeling in danger. It is this CRH hormone that starts an entire chain reaction, which ultimately gives us that energy kick when we are feeling stressed.

CRH does not affect our cells directly, and its influence usually is quite short. Instead, it uses intermediate messenger hormones secreted by glands that come into contact with CRH. One specific gland in this class is called the *pituitary* gland and is located just at the base of the brain.

The pituitary gland secrets yet another hormone, called *adrenocorticotropic hormone* (ACTH), which can travel much further through the bloodstream to influence nearly every organ. ACTH acts as the conductor of the stress response, transmitting the signal from the brain to all organs of the human body.

Although ACTH can act directly on certain organs, its primary role is to stimulate the secretion of yet another hormone, named *cortisol*, which has a much bigger impact on the function of human cells. This last hormone is secreted from the adrenal glands, situated right above our kidneys, and can travel through the bloodstream to influence many organs.

As you can see, the stress signal has to make its way through many layers, conducted through several intermediate hormones before it can affect our organs. Each one of these intermediate signaling hormones can be a cause for concern for our skin, as they can be mistaken by skin receptors to mean something not really intended by our brain.

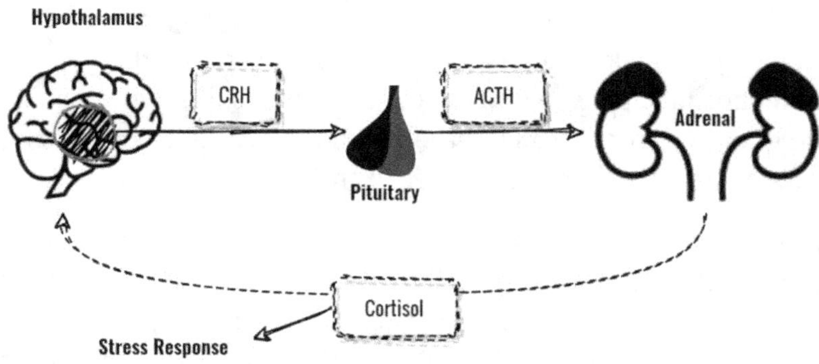

Figure 21 - Stress Response Axis

Although the exact path taken by the stress signal is not important, what is essential to note is that this information pipeline is a closed-loop and can regulate itself.

Both the hypothalamus and the anterior pituitary gland can sense if cortisol levels become too high and will dial down the production of their respective hormones if things get out of balance. This protects against prolonged stress activity, preventing long-term health degradation. This self-regulating stress response is kept in equilibrium most of the time, but it can be damaged if stress hormones are secreted for too long.

If we feel anxious for long periods, the body will eventually start to feel fatigued and will release less cortisol than it should. This protects organs from long-term exposure to stress, but it can also lead to other secondary health problems. Cortisol plays a crucial role in glucose metabolism, providing the energy our cells need to function correctly [392]. The longer the body is kept out of balance, the more severe the insensitivity to cortisol gets, and the longer it will take to heal once these abnormal feelings are stopped.

The skin is no different from any other organ in the human body. If stress hormones are released and circulate in the bloodstream, skin cells can choose to act upon these changes to support the flight-or-fight response. Because lipid and glucose production is a cornerstone that supports our ability to do intense physical activity, it shouldn't come as a surprise that some of these stress hormones mediate the process of generating lipids and sugars in the skin. In turn, this can interfere with the processes that create sebum, thus making pimples more likely to form.

During an experiment on sebum-producing cells, researchers found that lipid concentrations increased when CRH was applied directly to these cells. Lipid production increased by 60% when sebum cells were exposed to CRH [394]. Interestingly, this effect diminished with higher concentrations of CRH. This suggests that we would no longer feel these changes in our skin after passing a certain threshold of stress.

We now know that this effect is due to transcription factors that are fine-tuned to listen to the CRH hormone and which are present throughout our skin, including in the sebum-producing cells themselves [395]. These factors are aptly named CRH Receptor 1 and CRH Receptor 2 and can provide direct stimulation to sebum glands to increase their output.

As far as we can tell, these receptors have very little in common with other acne-inducing transcription factors that we've looked at in this book, including SREBP – the master regulator of lipids. Because of this, CRH and stress have a unique pathway that promotes acne, one which is not affected by our diet. If your acne is caused by stress, then changing your diet will likely not help due to these unique CRH receptors.

During the same study that found that lipid production is increased when cells come into contact with CRH, it was also found that CRH regulates the conversion of relatively inert androgens into testosterone. If you remember from previous chapters, certain androgens (male sex hormones) increase sebum production and are generally linked with a higher risk of getting acne [318]. For these androgen receptors to be activated, two preconditions must be met: the presence of the androgens hormones themselves and the inhibition of the FoxO1 transcription factor.

FoxO1 acts as a blocker of androgen receptors, as they mimic the shape of male sex hormones, allowing them to sit into these receptors. Although FoxO1 proteins can fit into androgen receptors, they don't fully activate them, but they do prevent other similar hormones from taking their intended place.

As an analogy, I'm sure you've experienced that certain keys can enter locks they weren't designed to open but can't exactly be used to turn the tumbler. Their shape matches that of the lock perfectly, but the groves on the key itself don't correctly set the unique set of pins inside the tumbler. Even if a key does fit inside a lock, that doesn't guarantee that you'll be able to open it fully. If, for some reason, such a key rusts inside the tumbler and you can't pry it out, then the lock is essentially closed forever, as you can't take the dud key out to add the correct one in.

This is the exact role FoxO1 plays with androgen receptors. Although FoxO1 can fit within these receptors, their structure is not entirely identical to that of androgens, meaning they can't turn these receptors on. But, once in this state, FoxOs prevent other androgens from entering these keyways and activating the receptors. We know that diet can force the migration of FoxOs outside the nucleus (thus preventing their acne-suppressive abilities), but it seems that CRH can also influence this aspect.

Besides insulin and IGF-1, we now know that FoxO1 has at least eight other antennas for various hormones and proteins that can be released in the bloodstream and which can disable this transcription factor. CRH is one of these signals [396].

It was found that CRH, through CRH Receptor 2, can suppress FoxO1 using the same signaling pathway used by insulin and IGF-1. This means that, besides the direct stimulation to FoxOs, CRH can potentially act on other transcription factors discussed in this book that can aggravate acne, such as mTOR. Although not fully tested, because the stress response affects common transcription factors to many acne-inducing pathways, it's very likely that CRH causes a cascade of changes that can exacerbate acne.

This problem can be compounded by the "stress eating" behavior many of us go through when dealing with anxiety-inducing events, which involves eating many "feel good" foods, such as fast carbs and fatty foods. These foods make us more likely to break out as they activate the transcription factors already mentioned in this book, including mTOR and SREBPs. However, if you add stress on top of that, this amplifies the entire effect, negating one of the few rheostats of these acne-inducing transcription factors.

What's more, CRH affects other mechanisms besides lipid production and androgen sensitivity that make pimples more likely. Specifically, CRH influences the immune system by changing the production of specific proteins that either promote or prevent inflammation [397]. This can potentially worsen acne once bacteria penetrates deep within the skin by making our skin more prone to inflammation.

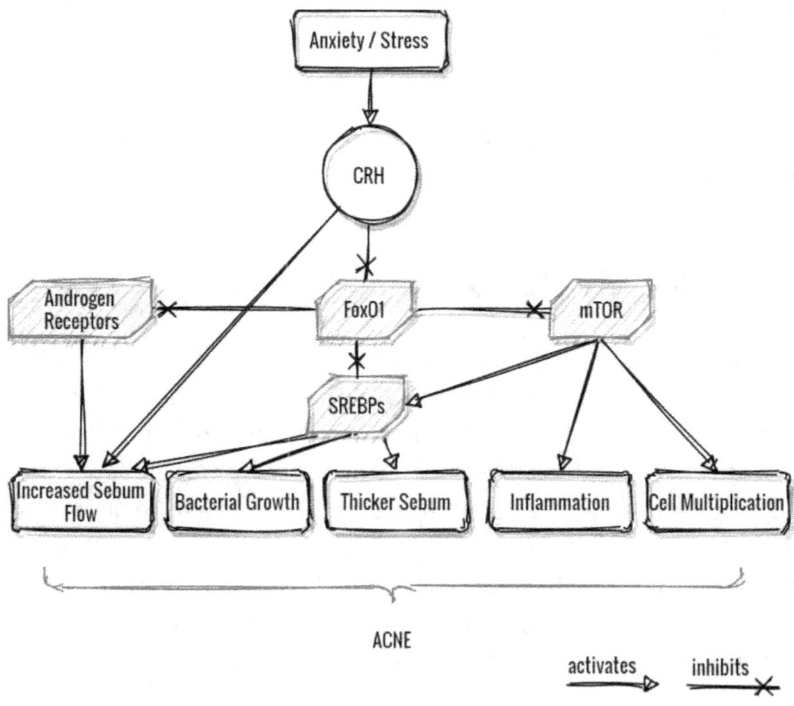

Figure 22 - Stress impact on acne

For these reasons, stress is particularly dangerous to our skin. It promotes the formation of pimples through its interaction with androgen receptors, it promotes sebum production, and it interferes with some central regulators of acne. All of these changes are induced through signals that are unique to stress and don't have any connection to any of the other acne-inducing factors looked at in this book.

Because of this, stress should be managed independently to help prevent acne, especially considering that it's a self-feeding fire. Having acne can lead to secondary mental health issues, including anxiety and stress, which can further worsen this disease. Once in this state, it can be challenging to break out, considering that very few dermatologists recommend seeking physiatric help alongside treating the primary disorder.

Yet, all is not without hope. If we acknowledge that acne is not just a superficial disease, we can make the first steps in breaking out of the loop.

Breaking the loop

Stress is of many types and has many causes – some of which are more easily treated than others. Acute stress is the heart-racing feeling we get when we are put under sudden dangerous, or unexpected situations. Acute stress only lasts for only a few hours to a few days and can be sometimes beneficial. We have all felt the last-minute panic when having to deliver a school or university project, alongside the super-human problem-solving abilities that come in this situation and help us stay focused longer. Short-term stress is beneficial to cognitive performance [398], which is why we're much more productive when in panic mode compared to normal. Because acute stress is brief, its impact on acne is also minimal.

Although these short-bursts of stressful feelings are beneficial, they can turn into long-term anxiety disorders (also known as chronic stress) if they persist for too long. If anxiety continues for a long time, this can have serious and long-lasting negative health effects.

How likely you are to develop chronic stress depends on many factors, including how prolonged the stressful events are, how varied the stressors are, and some genetic components that make us more likely to react badly to unwanted life events. Life happens, and most of these stressful situations are unavoidable. Despite this, we can teach ourselves how to respond better to these demanding events, such that they don't lead to more severe health problems. It's vital that we learn to deal with these situations well early on, as permanent feelings of anxiety can produce physical changes within our brain, making it much harder to break out of the loop once in this state.

If you repeat a task long enough, after some time, you will develop instincts that will help you complete the task faster, more accurately, and with less thought. Through this learning ability, we're able to develop highly complex skills, such as playing the piano, driving a car, or typing on a computer. For example, when you first start driving, you consciously have to think about which actions to take to get the car moving. Press the clutch pedal, press the break, make sure you are in neutral, start the engine, accelerate slightly, and let go of the clutch at the same time as you press the accelerator pedal. The first few times you try this, you'll most likely stall the engine, leading to frustration from you and your driving instructor. But, as you repeat these actions more and more, you'll get better at starting the car.

After some time, you won't give any thought to these steps – you just and in a car and go. If you try to explain to another beginner how to start a car, you'll likely have to think long and hard about the exact steps needed to get the car rolling, as everything you do is now done subconsciously. New connections have been made and strengthened in the neurons of your brain, which help you perform these tasks much more easily.

Although this learning process is beneficial in most situations, it can also create unwanted reflexes, making it difficult to break bad habits. These physical changes that occur in our brain can happen for undesirable behaviors as well, which can affect our ability to respond to stressful events [399].

You might have been put into a situation, sometime in your life, where you had to *unlearn* some bad behavior. If you've ever tried to give up smoking, you're likely well familiar with the cravings that come right after some daily routine event – like the morning cigarette break with a cup of coffee. Similarly, if you play a musical instrument, you might have inadvertently developed the wrong playing technique while learning to play, which is extremely hard to correct once you've become more proficient. It's hard to learn how to accomplish a complex task, but it's even harder to unlearn it. Yet, that is what you have to do if you want to treat chronic stress.

It's much more difficult to treat certain mental health issues (such as depression and anxiety) after you've had these conditions for a while. If given enough time, the unhelpful way we respond to unwanted life events becomes automatic and gradually moves into our subconscious. Once strong neural links are made to support these behaviors, it becomes much harder to break them. This is why the sooner you recognize the symptoms of anxiety, the easier it is to treat this disease.

Drugs are an obvious and popular choice for treating anxiety. The list of medications that can treat this disease is long, and some of them can even be bought without a prescription. Drugs are the most effective treatment method for anxiety disorders [400], making them an easy recommendation, especially if the condition is long-lasting. Yet, this type of treatment does come with some pretty significant drawbacks.

The most prescribed class of medications for anxiety, benzodiazepines, are addictive if taken long enough. If used occasionally or daily for a few weeks, benzodiazepines have a low risk of addiction. However, if used for more than a few weeks, this can increase the risk of abuse and dependence [401]. For this reason, anti-anxiety medications are only prescribed for a few weeks at a time, and you should not take them for longer than the prescribed treatment.

The real risk comes when benzodiazepines are combined with other medications, especially opioids. In the United States, 115 Americans die each day due to overdosing on opioids [402]. More than 30% of these overdoses also involve benzodiazepines.

Combining both drugs increases the dangers of overdosing, as both medications are sedatives, suppressing breathing and impairing cognitive functions. Studies have shown that people taking both drugs are at a higher risk of visiting the emergy room [403].

Even if we ignore the overdose and abuse potential of benzodiazepines, treating anxiety using drugs has another large disadvantage compared to alternative treatments. They do not teach you *how* to deal with stressful situations, and they do not help you unlearn destructive habits. Benzodiazepines only treat the superficial symptoms of anxiety but do not address the root cause of why people come to be in this situation.

You can treat a serious case of anxiety and depression using medications, but that does not mean you can't relapse into these negative thoughts after stopping treatment. If your only escape from these feelings is the pill, then you'll reach to it more often than you should, increasing the chances of abuse and overdose. What's more, this can create a learned behavior in and of itself. If you're feeling more stressed than usual, then you will crave the feel-good pills, even if you might not need them necessarily. That's why, even though drugs are the most effective short-term treatment for anxiety, they are no longer the gold standard [404] [405].

The current state-of-the-art treatment against anxiety disorders uses cognitive therapies, which teach you how to recognize these feelings early on and break the cycle without medication aid. These types of treatments address the root cause of anxiety disorders by teaching people how to deal with stressful situations in a more healthy manner. This minimizes the chances of relapsing and is a much better long-term treatment option with no side effects.

One of the most known forms of stress management techniques is *meditation*. If you're not aware of this technique, meditation is not simply the act of crossing your legs while chanting unintelligible words. Rather, it helps you block out random and worrying thoughts to focus your mind on your other senses, making you more aware of your surroundings and your body. In a way, it's a technique that teaches you to think about *nothing,* other than what our senses tell us at a specific moment in time. The end goal is to develop a way to cope with worry and anxiety by tuning out unwanted thoughts that can snowball into full-fledged anxiety disorders.

Practicing meditation is harder than it sounds. I challenge you to pause reading this book and spend the next 5 minutes thinking about *nothing.* If you've never done this before, you'll notice that your mind tends to drift to random thoughts – "I really have to go to the doctors next week," "I should get that noisy fan fixed," "why did I spend money on this stupid book." It takes practice to catch these thoughts and bring your mind back to a state of relaxation. If you're interested in trying these techniques yourself, a good place to start is at https://www.mindful.org/.

Meditation has been proven to be an effective stress management technique [406], and is easy to start with a plethora of apps that guide you through the experience. Despite this, meditation is not *the* most effective stress management technique; others have been proven more successful [404] [405]. Because of this, meditation is no longer the most recommended stress-management treatment. Instead, *cognitive behavioral therapy* (CBT) is the first recommendation given to people with anxiety.

CBT is a class of mental exercises that improve the general mental health of patients by challenging and changing unhelpful thoughts.

Traditional therapies for mental disorders, such as psychoanalysis, seek the root cause of stressful feelings by discussing traumatizing and unwanted life events. Once the cause of the distress is known, then the patient can work towards correcting the behavior.

CBT takes a different approach, whereby it doesn't care about the root cause of the stressful feelings. Instead, it takes active steps to catch and correct negative thoughts early on. This way, you're no longer conditioned to feel depressed or anxious when life is particularly tough. Instead of treating just a single traumatizing event, you learn how to deal with challenging situations in general, protecting your future from further traumatizing situations.

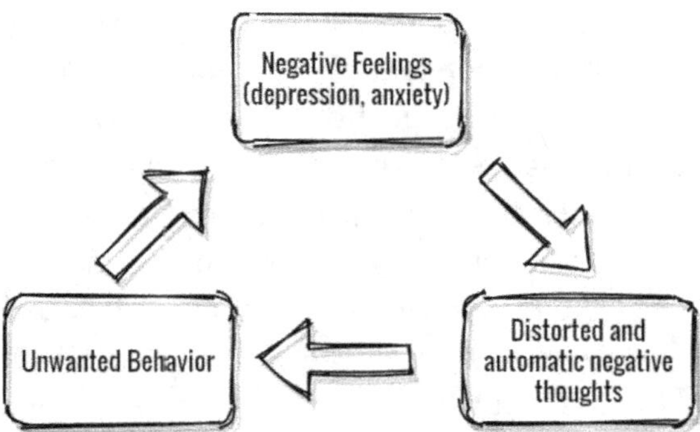

Figure 23 - Influence of feelings on thoughts

CBT is most effective when the mental disorder persists for a long time. People who are chronically depressed will tend to assign blame to themselves, deepening the depressive state. Automatic thoughts, such as "I am worthless," "other people aren't as careless like me," or "everybody hates me for making this mistake"; surface even in trivial situations. CBT trains people to recognize these unhelpful thoughts and to put them in a critical light.

The same is true for anxiety-inducing thoughts, such as "if I fail this exam, this is the end of my life," "what if I get fired for making this mistake," or "I'm certain I will develop cancer by my 40s". CBT teaches patients how to detect these unhelpful thoughts, objectively assess them, and create concrete steps that can be taken to alleviate the trigger.

CBT therapies are based on just two simple techniques:

1. **Identify distorted views**. This can be especially hard if they become automatic and part of learned behavior. It usually takes a specialist to point them out to us.
2. **Objectively assess the situation and change the distorted thoughts accordingly**.

One specialized form of CBT developed specifically to manage stress is called *Pythagorean Self-Awareness Intervention (PSAI).* It is more a form of introspection of one's day, whereby people explore events that occur recently, objectively assess them, and then devise concrete actions if the outcome was undesirable. By evaluating one's actions and creating tangible plans to correct any wrongdoings, we're reducing the worry that is usually associated with these events. After all, anxiety and stress are a way of planning for the future and for the unknown – albeit in a very inefficient way. Once we take care of the unknown and create a concrete plan to alleviate some of these problems, then we can mitigate the worry we feel as well.

Concretely, if you're planning on applying PSAI at home, you should set aside some time right before bed to go through the following steps in order:

1. First, recall and note all major events which happened during the respective day in the exact order in which they occurred.
2. Review each one of these events by checking what you did wrong, what you did right, and if there was anything else about this event you wish you could have done. Remember to be objective during this review and detach yourself from any emotions (positive or negative) that you might have.
3. During the next morning, after you're reviewed the findings from the previous night, make concrete plans and goals for the current day.
4. Follow these steps, both in the morning and in the evening, each and every day for a minimum of 3-4 weeks.

> It takes time to re-wire the brain, so don't be discouraged
> if improvements can't be seen from the first few days.

The methodology mentioned above is pretty slimmed down, and if you're serious about applying it in the long term, you're sure to find more detailed guides online. However, all PSAI methodologies are based on the same basic steps: first, analyze what went right and what went wrong for a given day; and then make concrete plans on what to improve the following day. This technique is also helpful if you have frequent sleepless nights, as it has been shown to help insomniacs [407]. And, more relevant to us, PSAI has also been shown to help with acne.

To see if PSAI can treat acne, an experiment was created with a simple premise: take 30 women, split them into two groups – one used as a control, and one which applies PSAI daily – and then measure any changes in acne severity following an 8-week trial. The patients who applied PSAI did so in two stages: in the evening, they noted down the events of the previous day objectively; while in the morning, they thought of concrete actions that should be taken to address the events of the previous day.

On average, patients enrolled in the PSAI group did see an improvement in acne severity. Out of a total of 15 women in the intervention group, 5 of them were completely cured. What's more, out of the 9 initial cases of moderate to severe acne, all improved to either light acne or completely cured (Figure 24 - Changes in acne severity following PSAI treatment) [408]. Granted, this was a tiny study, but it's nonetheless evidence that by better managing our response to stressful life events, we're able to improve our acne as well.

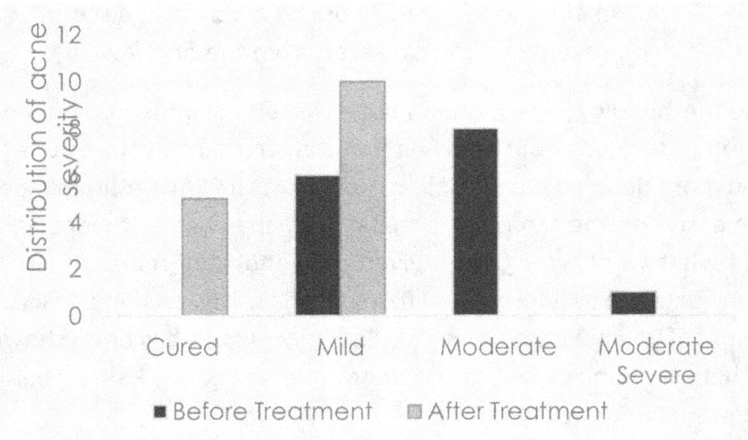

Figure 24 - Changes in acne severity following PSAI treatment

This idea that acne can be improved by managing secondary mental disorders is still relatively new, hence why there haven't been that many studies to date on this topic. More so, although 30% to 60% of dermatological patients suffer from some kind of psychiatric disorder [409], relatively few such cases are detected by medical physicians and directed for treatment [410].

Although these concepts are relatively new, they are growing in awareness, even leading to a special branch of skincare named *psychodermatology,* which blends conventional medical treatments for skin diseases with psychological care to achieve the maximum results for both conditions. Patients that follow these types of treatments report higher success rates compared to conventional therapies [411]. Such clinics are still rare, so you'd likely be better off visiting specialists for psychiatric disorders yourself, considering that dermatologists still largely ignore this aspect of acne.

Overall, it's clear to see that acne, depression, and anxiety and closely intertwined. It's also apparent that acne is not just a disease of our bodies but can equally affect our mental well-being. Because this machinery is so complex, it's also hard to treat.

We can't fix these components in isolation without looking at the entire ensemble in its entirety. We should also not rely only on dermatologists and medical professionals to guide us through these problems because, at the end of the day, each practitioner specializes in a single domain of medicine, while acne seems to affect a wide area of human health. We should recognize these secondary health problems ourselves and seek professional help before they become long-lasting psychiatric disorders that affect our job security, academic performance, social relationships, and general wellbeing.

CHAPTER SUMMARY

- Acne is known to cause severe secondary mental health issues, such as anxiety and depression. These psychological problems can persist long after acne is cured, leading to a decreased quality of life in those affected. It is important to recognize depression and anxiety early in acne patients and treat these secondary illnesses accordingly.

- Chronic stress is also thought to cause acne. The hormones that cause the fight-or-flight response also affect the skin, promoting inflammation, sebum production, and activation of androgen receptors. This pathway is separate from other dietary factors looked at so far in this book and needs to be treated separately.

- Both acne and anxiety are caught in a feedback loop, where one causes the other, amplifying both diseases. This makes it much harder to break out of the loop, especially if both diseases persist for a long time.

- Medication is the most effective treatment option for combating chronic stress, yet there is no evidence to suggest that treating stress this way will also cure acne.

- Alternative treatments for managing anxiety, such as cognitive behavioral therapy, are effective in reducing stress and in improving acne.

SMOKING

Tobacco remains one of the largest killers in the world. Despite the constant campaigning by governments and health organizations, tobacco still kills 8 million people each year. Of these deaths, 1.2 million are the result of second-hand smoking [412]. The World Health Organisation called tobacco smoking the "biggest public health threat the world has ever faced" [413], making it the largest preventable cause of disease and premature death. Smoking increases the chances of dying from heart disease and stroke by 2 to 4 times and is responsible for 90% of lung cancer deaths and 80% of chronic obstructive pulmonary disease deaths [414]. Tobacco usage can cause damage in nearly every organ of the human body, including the esophagus, kidneys, lungs, stomach, pancreas, liver, upper respiratory tract, and many more [415]. Seeing as smoking is so damaging to the human body, it's not a stretch of the imagination to assume that smoking can also harm our skin.

Research on the link between smoking and acne is surprisingly conflictual. About a third of past experiments on this topic show that tobacco usage does cause acne [416] [307] [417] [418] [419], another third indicates that smoking actually helps acne [420] [421] [422] [423] [424], while the rest show no connection between the two [308] [425] [426] [427] [428] [429]. This conflictual data indicates that there is a more complex interaction between tobacco and our skin. Some of the effects of smoking are likely harmful, but some might actually be protective against acne.

These conflictual effects likely come from the main active ingredient in cigarettes, namely nicotine – a potent neuro-stimulating substance. We can't produce nicotine ourselves, and it has no real use for us. The reason why it has this calming effect (and why it is so addictive) is more coincidental and can be explained by the real reason plants secrete this substance – to kill.

In nature, nicotine is produced as a toxin by some plants to deter predators. Nicotine targets a set of receptors named *nicotinic acetylcholine receptors* (nAChRs) that are present throughout our body and are used in a wide range of bodily functions. Normally, another hormone that is produced naturally in humans stimulates these receptors. However, nicotine tricks our body and these receptors into thinking the intended hormone is being released, creating unwanted side effects.

nAChRs generally help with tasks relating to sustaining life and escaping from predators, such as muscle contraction and supporting the autonomic nervous system. This is why, after we smoke a cigarette, we get that relaxing feeling throughout our muscles. Nicotine over-stimulates the nAChR receptors that are present in muscle tissue, making us feel more relaxed. However, for some organisms, this soothing effect can be overwhelming and, in some instances, even fatal. Small insects and parasites are particularly sensitive to nicotine, hence why Mother Nature has given some plants the ability to secrete this toxin.

Nicotine is so effective as a neurotoxin that it was widely used as a pesticide until the mid-1960s until better and safer alternatives were found [430]. Thankfully, humans and most complex organisms have evolved safety mechanisms against nicotine [430], meaning this substance is harmless to us in low dosages.

Over many thousands of years, humans have developed a selective filter against nicotine in muscle cells, whereby the relaxing effect is negated almost entirely. The nicotine receptors in muscle tissue are 50 times less sensitive than the ones found in our neurons [430], which is why nicotine has a much more pronounced effect on the brain than any other organ. Evolution has given us ways to neutralize nicotine's life-threatening effects but has still left us open to the calming properties through our neuron receptors. Yet, our brain and muscles aren't the only organs that have nicotine receptors. Our skin has them as well, which gives us a hint as to why smoking can affect acne.

One group of researchers analyzed the skin properties of smokers and non-smokers in the hopes of finding why smoking can be beneficial to some acne patients but detrimental to others. The researchers analyzed the skin of randomly selected women by looking at the composition of the sebum between smokers and non-smokers.

The researchers found that there is a significant difference in the ingredients of sebum between the two groups, whereby the sebum collected from the smokers had half the concentration of certain antioxidants compared to the non-smoking group. Having lower concentrations of antioxidants means that something is causing more oxidative stress to the skin, depleting the reserves of these nutrients. Without antioxidants reserves, the skin is more vulnerable to other sources of oxidations, including pollution and UV radiation.

Besides lower concentrations of antioxidants, the researchers also found that the sebum of smokers contained fewer squalene compounds and more squalene oxidants. It seems that smoking can convert squalene into oxides of this substance, which are likely the source of the oxidative damage observed in the skin [431].

From previous chapters, we've seen that oxides of squalene can be highly comedogenic (can cause pore blockages) and can significantly increase the likelihood of developing pimples [432]. Notably, these compounds were found to induce inflammation, promote pore blockages, and increase the rate at which skin cells are created and die [360] [208].

In one experiment, researchers shot UV light at normal squalene to make oxidized squalene and see if this new mixture will negatively influence the surrounding skin. This type of radiation has enough energy to change the very chemical composition of squalene, mimicking the changes we would see from smoking or when we are exposed to air pollution. In the end, the researchers found that regions of the skin that were exposed to oxidized squalene had more blocked pores, and these blockages were larger in diameter. This effect became more pronounced with higher concentrations of squalene oxides. At the highest measured levels, pore blockages were twice as large compared to regions with normal squalene levels [433].

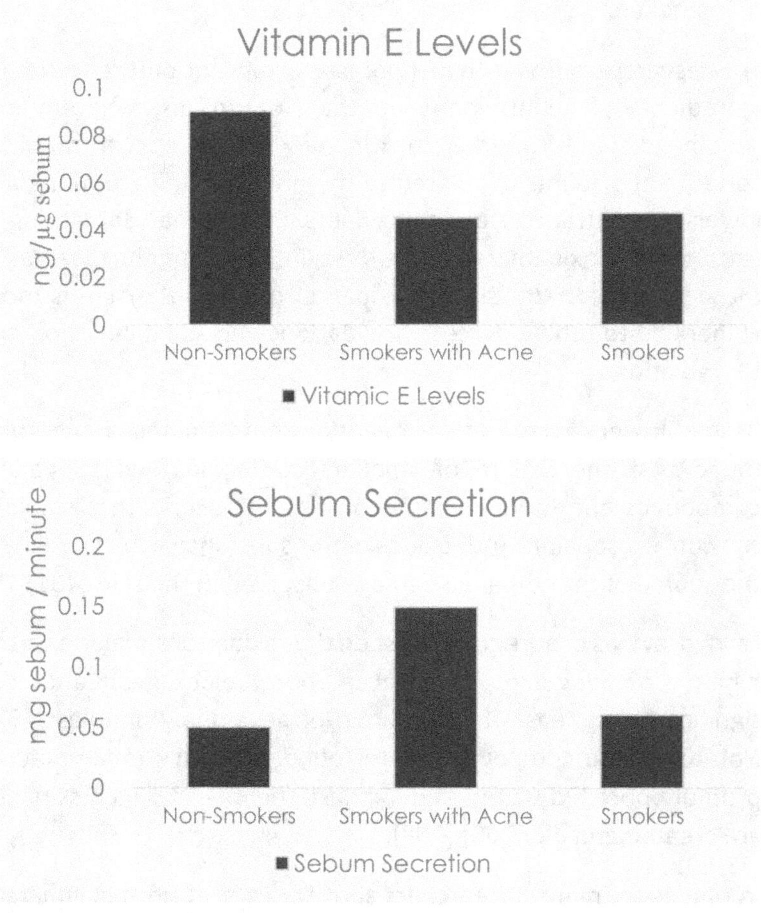

Figure 25 - Smoking effect on sebum

We now know that cigarette smoke can also oxidize squalene, potentially aggravating acne through the previously discussed effects. In-vitro tests have shown that squalene gets converted into squalene oxides if exposed to cigarette smoke [434].

A group of researchers exposed the forearm of some patients to cigarette smoke and then measured any chemical changes that might have happened to the sebum in this region. After a 10 minute exposure, the conversion process between squalene and its oxides increased significantly and stayed elevated many tens of minutes after the initial exposure [434]. The researchers attributed these changes to some potent free radicals present in cigarette smoke, namely tar and some other gases [435]. The researchers also suggested that antioxidants (such as those found in oolong tea) can prevent these chemical changes if applied to the skin.

This squalene transformation likely explains why we see conflictual data on smoking and acne. Those who smoke predominantly outside are not as exposed to cigarette smoke as those that do so inside. Because of this, the squalene of outdoor smokers gets less oxidized, protecting the smokers against this type of acne. If you do smoke and plan on continuing to do so (despite all the other health risks associated with this habit), making sure you smoke in a well-ventilated space will help prevent acne.

Even so, smoking outside is not a guaranteed way of preventing acne, as this habit causes other changes within our body that can make us more likely to break out.

Experiments have shown that certain acne-inducing transcription factors are sensitive to nicotine and other carcinogens found in cigarette smoke [396]. Notably, it was found that the same antennas used by FoxO1 to detect body nutrition and stress levels are also sensitive to nicotine and other chemicals found in cigarette smoke [396].

If you remember from previous chapters, FoxO1 is a crucial regulator of sebum production, cell multiplication, and inflammation. It interacts with other transcription factors that are heavily tied to acne, namely mTOR and SREBPs, acting as a rheostat to various factors that can cause pimples. Because smoking interferes with this central regulator, this habit can likely induce changes in our body that promote acne, namely increased sebum production, cell multiplication, and immune system changes. Throughout this book, we've seen that our diet generally drives these internal changes, but it seems that smoking can also interfere with normal cell function.

What's more, the AChRs receptors that respond to nicotine were found in maturing sebum-producing cells [436] and in cells that form the outer layer of skin pores. When these receptors are activated, they increase the rate at which skin cells multiply and die, thus providing raw material for new pore blockages to form [437]. These effects were found in concentrations of nicotine that are entirely possible through regular smoking [438].

All in all, the changes brought onto our skin by smoking are incredibly damaging. We've seen this vice promotes unwanted changes from direct contact between cigarette smoke and our skin and through internal changes that make us more prone to breaking out.

Considering that cigarettes have such a devastating effect on our skin, why then does some research shows that smoking can benefit us?

The answer to this likely comes from the interaction between smoking and our immune system. The protective effect doesn't come because we no longer get pimples but because our skin doesn't react as severely to pore blockages.

The health dangers of smoking are well known, but what is less known is that smoking can sometimes lower the chances of developing certain diseases. Smokers have lower incidence rates for Parkinson's disease, farmer's lung, uterine fibroids, pigeon breeders' disease, and others [439]. What most of these diseases have in common is that they are caused by excessive inflammation in some organs or are tied in some way to inflammation. Smoking helps prevent these diseases by dialing down our immune system, thus reducing inflammation and any subsequent damage to our organs.

Nicotine was found to inhibit the function of T cells (a type of white blood cell that plays a vital role in the immune response), thus preventing the immune system from functioning correctly [440]. Because acne is also primarily caused by excessive inflammation, it's plausible that nicotine's anti-inflammatory properties can help alleviate this disease. Although smoking indirectly causes inflammation through the oxidation of squalene, this effect could be counteracted by the suppressive effect on the immune system. This is likely why some people report improvements in acne from smoking. Their immune system is so damaged that it can no longer fight against the acne-inducing bacteria that seeps into our skin.

Overall, although there are some probable advantages to smoking, the negative health implications far outweigh these benefits. If reducing inflammation is your aim, then there are other, safer ways to accomplish this. For example, you can consume fruits and vegetables rich in antioxidants, which were proven to reduce inflammation [441], or you can take anti-inflammatory drugs (such as ibuprofen or aspirin). The added benefit to these alternative treatments is that they have been shown to decrease the chances of developing other inflammation-driven diseases, including Parkinson's [442] [443], without any of the health risks brought by smoking.

In the end, cigarette smoking remains one of the largest killers in modern society, with severe adverse effects on our skin. Because the marginal benefits brought by smoking can be had with safer alternatives, you should still avoid this habit at all costs.

CHAPTER SUMMARY

- Nicotine is a toxin used by some plants to deter predators. Although humans have evolved defenses against these life-threatening effects, we still have nicotine receptors in some organs, including our skin.

- Smoking depletes antioxidant reserves from our skin and promoted the conversion of squalene into squalene oxides. This mixture makes the skin more prone to pore blockages and inflammation.

- Some people report improvements in acne while smoking. These protective effects come from the suppressive properties of nicotine over our immune system, making the skin less prone to inflammation. Even so, there are safer alternatives that reduce inflammation (such as fruits, legumes, and some drugs), meaning smoking should still be avoided.

PUBERTY AND HORMONES

Adolescence can be both a period of wonder but also one of confusion. Most might remember these days with fondness, even going so far as saying that it was the best years of their life. However, there's no denying that the changes that occur in our bodies during this time can be confusing and even scary if you're not prepared.

Our voices deepen, hair starts to grow in unexpected places, our height grows unusually quickly, and fat and muscle begin to deposit in places that make us look more like adults rather than children. We don't change just physically, but also in our mental abilities. Although we don't gain brain mass during adolescence (by age 6, the brain already has 90% of the mass of an adult human [444]), complex changes occur in the structure and connections between neurons that cultivate emotional maturity and improved cognition. By the time we are 15, thinking abilities are comparable to those of adults. This explosion of cognitive capabilities is thanks, in part, to improvements to memory, abstract thinking, the speed at which we think, and our attention span. These rapid changes that occur only in a few years help us transition from children into adults, making us unrecognizable to our parents and friends. Yet, not all changes are beneficial.

Most of us have experienced traumatizing incidents during high school, either from bullying or from embarrassing events. Psychologists define this transitional phase between childhood and adolescence as one in which antisocial behavior starts [445]. Although many factors can influence antisocial tendencies — including a lack of supervision from parents — in the most extreme cases, it can lead to peer bullying and aggressive behavior towards others.

It's not surprising to learn that teenagers start to develop anxiety and depressive disorders during this time [446]. And, although the highest rates of mental illness are found in our 30s and 40s, adolescence is when these illnesses first set in. Some of these conditions start as early as 11 years old, especially phobias and separation anxiety disorders [446]. Young girls are especially susceptible to these changes, being twice as likely to experience depression or anxiety episodes compared to young boys [446]. During this transitional phase of our life, we are extremely sensitive to traumatizing events that can set the stage for long-term social phobias. This is why peer bullying is so damaging during this time and why acne can be so harmful to normal social development. The fact that acne is more common during these critical years, which gives more opportunities for peer bullying, certainly doesn't help prevent these traumas.

If you're reading this book and have acne, you likely got your first pimples during adolescence. Why would nature play such a cruel joke on us when we are the most vulnerable and needing social connections is anyone's guess. It seems counter-intuitive that Mother Nature would cripple us in these crucial moments of our life in a way that hinders our academic performances, creates long-lasting social phobias, and burdens us in our transition into adulthood.

It might seem that the acne we get while growing up is unavoidable, a kind of "rite of passage" into adulthood. Yet, this might not be necessarily so. In this final chapter, we'll explore if the acne we get while growing up is as inescapable as it might appear, to put the last piece of the puzzle together and get a complete picture of how acne works and what we can do to prevent it. These final pages are dedicated to understanding why acne is so much more common in our early years and how this interplays with everything we've learned so far.

Do teenagers get more acne?

Yes.

Numerous studies have shown that you're much more likely to have acne if you are within a certain age range, particularly in your late teens. It's well established that age is the best predictor of acne. The years you've lived have a stronger link with acne than your diet, sex, genetic factors, smoking habits, and almost everything else you can imagine. If you reach the age of 19, you have an 80-95% chance of having acne at least once in your life. However, children aged nine and younger have an almost 0% chance of developing pimples [447] [448].

Although this fact is pretty well known, what's striking is exactly how quickly your risk increases after a certain age and how quickly it drops once you reach early adulthood. Although the highest acne rates are found in people aged 15-19, as you reach your late 20s, your chances of still having acne drop to a quarter. If you're in your young adult years, you have a 64% chance of still having acne [418]. However, as you move into adulthood, acne rates drop sharply. Only 3-5% of people between 40 and 49 continue to have acne [449].

This sharp decrease in acne rates explains why there are so many self-reported remedies for acne. The internet is filled with bizarre treatments for pimples, ranging from banana peels, ice, a good soaking in your own urine, snail slime, and window cleaner [450]. Even without a medical degree, I trust that you can see why all such "treatments" likely do more harm than good.

We have so many wacky remedies because acne will eventually go away on its own, an event that might coincide with someone testing one of these therapies. Acne also naturally fluctuated with time, even if you might still be at an age at risk of developing pimples. Your diet might change, you might go through more stressful events, or your hormones might fluctuate due to menstrual cycles or some other diseases (e.g., PCOS). These unusual remedies might overlap with a period when acne heals itself for some time, leading people to believe that the treatment actually worked. But, until these treatments are put through rigorous scientific testing, I would avoid them and instead stick to tried-and-tested treatments. I would definitely like to see how some poor scientist has to convince acne patients to soak their face into urine daily for 12 weeks.

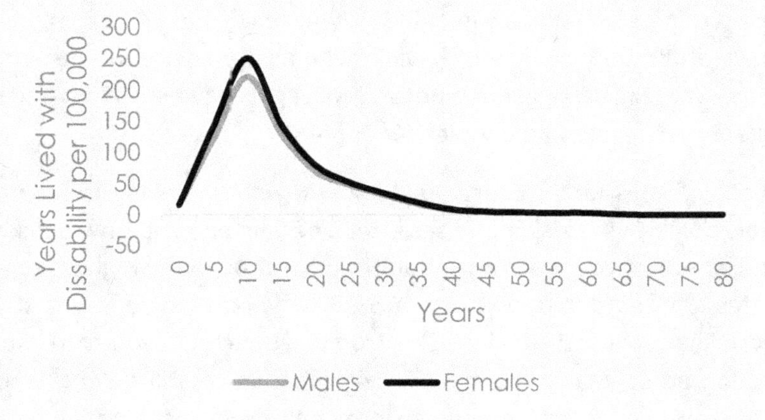

Figure 26 - Acne rates by age

The fact that acne naturally clears itself after a certain age is undoubtedly good news for most. If your acne is not too severe, a straightforward option to treat this condition would be to simply wait it out, as your skin will naturally tend to get better over time.

Despite this good news, recent research is beginning to show some worrying trends about this aspect. Since around the mid-90s, scientists have observed that puberty tends to start earlier than usual, potentially interfering with acne's natural course [451].

A Danish study found that between 1993 and 2008, the average age at which puberty hits has decreased by approximately 95 days [451]. The earlier puberty kicks in, the earlier acne develops, and the more we have to live with this disease.

Because of these changes in puberty timing, dermatology clinics have seen an uptick in acne patients as young as 8 to 9 years old [452]. Children are significantly less mature at this age, which can lead to more bullying, teasing, and life-long social phobias. Traumas experienced early in life create permanent physical changes in the brain [453] that make you more likely to develop mental health disorders later in life, such as depression or PTSD [454]. It's unknown why we see this early onset of puberty, but researchers speculate that better nutrition and increased obesity rates are to blame.

Although it's well established that adolescents have a higher prevalence of acne, the reason why is not fully known.

We know that sebum plays a vital role in acne development and that hair follicles start producing sebum only after the age of 8 to 10 [455]. Before that age, pore blockages can form, but without sebum to host the acne-causing bacteria, these blockages rarely grow into full-blown inflamed acne. Even so, the late development of sebum-producing glands is likely not the cause of the initial wave of acne. Instead, it's the first time we see the manifestation of an imbalance in our body and our skin.

Similar to how the sun is shining its light even when we don't see it during the night, the underlying problems that cause acne can still exist even if there is no sebum. After all, acne usually disappears as we enter our adult years, but we continue to produce sebum throughout our life. Only after 50 years or so do we start seeing a decline in sebum rates, but the changes are not drastic even then. By the time we hit 80, sebum production drops by only about 30% from middle age [456]. It's clear that sebum production is not the only factor to blame for the acne we get during adolescence.

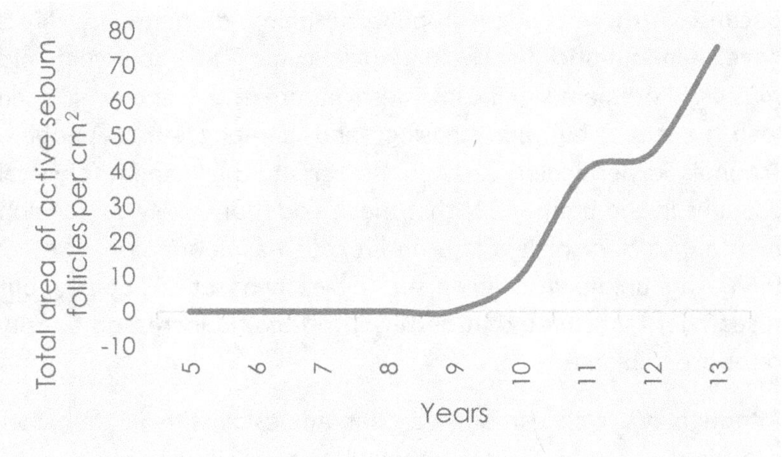

Figure 27 - Number of hair folicles that secrete sebum

It's also important to remember that not everyone develops acne in their teenage years – some, not at all. The tribes that we discussed at the beginning of this book – Aché and Kitavan tribes – reported no acne cases across all age ranges. Of the 300 Kitavan young adults aged 15 – 25 who participated in the study, none had developed acne throughout the examination period that lasted 843 days [1]. As people from these tribes have similar physiology to Westerners, sebum is clearly not the main culprit that causes acne. Instead, some other agent disrupts our skin's health, which can only manifest itself once skin pores start to secrete sebum.

To find the actual cause, we have to look at some other changes that happen in our bodies during this transitional phase of our life. But, unlike sebum, we have to find something that only happens in early adulthood and which abruptly disappears when we reach our 20s. One obvious place to start is the bodily system that drives the growth we see during adolescence. Our body grows in mass and height from birth all the way up to our late teens. This timeline is suspiciously similar to that of acne, pointing towards a link between the two.

A time of growth

If we look at the progression of our growth, from the moment we are born up until adulthood, we might think that this development is continuous and gradual. In this period, we get taller, we become smarter with each passing year, our reflexes and reasoning become better, and our muscles and physical strength increase. Although these changes might seem progressive at first, we really pass through multiple development stages, each with its own characteristics.

In infancy, brain maturity happens at an incredible rate, whereby 90% of brain growth happens before kindergarten. In the first year of our life, the brain doubles in size, which is why the experiences felt in infancy are crucial to our success throughout our life.

In contrast, the latter stages of our development are characterized by physical changes to our bodies. Although we grow in height and size throughout our childhood, we see a significant growth spurt only in the later years. Likewise, besides growth in mass, our bodies also go through changes that accentuate our biological sex. If you're a young boy, testicles develop, your voice deepens, and the first few facial hairs start to appear. Similarly, if you're a young girl, breasts become bigger, and menstruation begins.

For these reasons, puberty is characterized by body growth and sex differentiation. Growth signals make us gain stature, while the sex differentiation signal accentuates the differences between men and women. Both of these aspects are also relevant to this book. The way our body decides when and how much to grow can also affect acne.

When we're around two years old, our height measures about 80cm to 90cm. From there, we grow, like clockwork, about 5cm in height each year, reaching our peak during late puberty. We stop growing at ages 17 to 19, but the peak growth rate is reached much sooner than this, at around ages 12 to 14. Coincidentally, this is also the peak age when we see the highest number of acne cases, pointing to a link between acne and body growth.

Seeing as we don't continue growing after a certain age, there must be a hidden signal our body uses to dictate when to grow and when to stop growing. What better way to transmit this signal to the 30,000,000,000,000 cells in our body than to use *hormones?*

Remember that hormones are a distinct class of signaling molecules that are secreted by various organs and which can travel throughout our body. Nerve fibers are one way to transmit information between cells, but they require a long cable to be stretched from the transmitter to the receiver. Although very accurate, it's not practical to lay such nerve fibers to all of our cells. For this reason, we have evolved a secondary way of communication between organs, one which trades precision for efficiency.

The human nerve network is similar to how early telegraph systems used to work. To transmit information between two people, a long strand of wire was laid out between a person writing a message and the receiver. The telegraph operator would input words in an encoded format, which were transmitted instantly over the wire tens of kilometers away. To support the growing cities of the 19th century, thousands of kilometers of such telegraph wire were laid out. Although this communication system only really took off in the United States, at its peak, 200 million messages were sent in total [457]. Telegrams were highly successful, especially considering that the alternative was horse-delivered messages or optical flag systems.

However, although telegrams revolutionized communication at that time, they did suffer from one major flaw. It required a physical cable to be laid out between two operators. This meant that it was difficult to add this communication system in moving vehicles or in masses to every household.

The telegraph was very accurate, as you transmitted your message to a single person. Still, it was impractical if you wanted to send information over long distances or to many people all at once. When wireless communication came along, it solved long-distance communication as information can now be broadcasted using electromagnetic waves that can travel unimpeded over vast distances. However, this innovation also reduced precision – anyone can listen to these communications and hear your message. With wireless transmission, it became much harder to send messages to just a single person and even harder to do so in a way that can't easily be decoded by other people listening on the same channel.

Hormones suffer from the same problem – they are inaccurate. It's near impossible to control who gets a particular message. It's up to the receiver to decide if they want to act upon a specific action, and the chances of miscommunication are high. It's for these reasons that the signals governing growth and sex differentiation can also affect acne. The hormones that control bodily changes during puberty also interplay with skin cells in unintended ways, increasing the odds of pimples forming.

The primary conductor of growth in the human body is a hormone called *human growth hormone (HCH)*. As its name suggests, HCH manages cell reproduction and growth, and it's produced in higher quantities during early childhood. It promotes organ development (especially muscle tissue), stimulates fat usage, and generally ramps up the factories that produce glucose and energy to sustain these demanding processes.

HCH stays relatively elevated throughout our life, slowly diminishing as we age, leading some to speculate that the gradually declining levels of HCH are responsible for our aging. For this reason, some have called HCH the "fountain of youth" and is commonly marketed as a drug that prevents aging and which helps with athletic performance. Despite its popularity among athletes, there is limited evidence to suggest that taking HCH supplements has any effect on physical strength or in preventing age-related diseases [458].

Even though HCH is the primary regulator of growth in the human body, it is likely not the most significant driver of acne. HCH levels peak when we are born and decline as we age, even during puberty. Because acne rates peak much later than HCH levels, the correlation between the two does not look strong. However, HCH is not the only hormone that controls cell growth and reproduction; there are others. HCH might be the main conductor, but it has subordinates who help direct the growth signal to intended organs. One such hormone is *Insulin-like Growth Factor 1* (IGF-1), which came up quite a few times during this book. Many of the effects of HCH on body growth are actually mediated by IGF-1.

Compared to HCH, IGF-1 has a much more pronounced effect on body development. Besides muscle growth, IGF-1 also stimulates bone strengthening, protein synthesis, blood vessel growth, and others [459]. Deficiencies in IGF-1 are associated with diseases that stunt growth, in which the body does not develop fully before reaching adulthood.

On the other end of the spectrum, IGF-1 has also emerged as a central player in aging and age-related diseases. In rodent and human tests, low levels of IGF-1 were associated with increased lifespan, lower cognitive decline, and suppressed cancer growth [460]. This recent data suggest that IGF-1 must be kept in constant balance for optimal health; too little IGF-1 and the body does not develop fully in weight and in height; too much IGF-1 and aging is accelerated. Yet, having an imbalance in IGF-1 serum levels does not affect only growth and aging. More relevant to us, abnormally large quantities of IGF-1 are also thought to trigger acne.

Unlike HCH (which peaks during early childhood), IGF-1 levels are highest during adolescence, at the ages of 13 to 15 [461]. This is also the age at which we see the highest rates of acne in children.

If we overlap a graph showing IGF-1 levels broken down by age with a chart for acne rates, we see that the peaks of the two are surprisingly similar (see Figure 28 - Link between IGF-1 levels and acne). When the IGF-1 signal is the strongest, we also experience the highest growth rate and the most pimples.

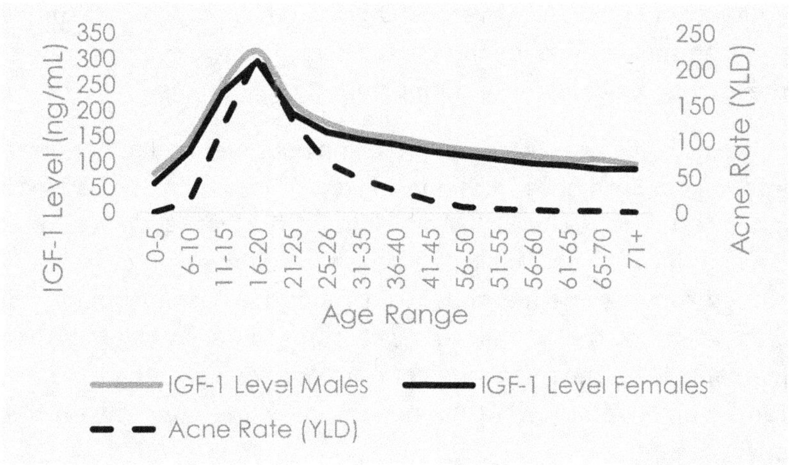

Figure 28 - Link between IGF-1 levels and acne [668]

IGF-1 does not directly cause organ growth, and it is purely used to send information from the secreting organ to various cells within our body. IGF-1 does not even enter our cells to affect gene transcription. Instead, it binds to receptors on the surface of cell membranes that relay this signal to internal transcription factors and other cell components. Because of this, the IGF-1 message can still be intercepted and manipulated, giving us a way to control the negative health implications brought by this hormone.

The act of growing is a constant balance between prosperity and survival. Similar to how you don't start building an annex to your house if you lack enough bricks, cells don't start multiplying and growing if there aren't enough nutrients to support this process. In previous chapters, we've seen that mTOR is the controller that senses whether the body is getting sufficient nutrients before allowing cell systems to act on growth signals. mTOR has many antennas that sense the state the body is in; some look for amino acids that indicate f we are well fed, while others respond to growth signals. We've previously seen that insulin can provide the growth signal to mTOR, tricking cells into thinking that they should multiply and grow. However, mTOR is also tunned to listed to the IGF-1 hormone, meaning this transcription factor can also regulate the growth we experience during puberty.

It's easy to see how the acne induced by our diet and puberty are interlinked. Both have the same triggers. The acne we experience in adolescence is caused by an influx of hormones that help us develop into adults. While the acne that happens later in life is caused by the same hormones, but artificially raised through our diet. Even so, the pimples we get during puberty are still not inescapable, as the signals we get from our bodies during this time can be amplified by what we eat and how we interact with the environment.

Our body naturally secretes growth hormones that help us develop into fully functioning adults during our early years. Under normal circumstances, this process is beneficial and indeed vital to our health. mTOR supports this process by ensuring organ growth only happens when we are not deprived of essential nutrients. It makes sense for this master regulator of growth to listen to both growth hormones and nutritional state. However, mTOR and other similar transcription factors are tuned for maximum efficiency when these hormones are within narrow limits. If we introduce elements in our diet that makes the body secrete too many growth and nutrient signals, then our survival systems are overloaded and are put out of balance.

We've evolved these systems when proteins were scarce, and sugars only came in the form of occasional fruits with a low glycemic load. Back then, it didn't matter if growth hormones were detected by skin cells because it wasn't possible to go over the limit with the usual diet. However, with the increase in consumption of refined carbohydrates, meats, and milk, the human body over-produces growth hormones past the point we can deal with naturally. The growth signals we emit during puberty are superimposed by those emitted, inadvertently, by our diet. As a result, the governors of growth are over-stimulated, producing unintended consequences that are harmful to our skin and our general health. Puberty is not to blame for our acne, but rather "super puberty" that is artificially created and magnified by our unnatural diets.

It might seem like we've cracked the code for acne now that we've found the relationship between pubescent and adult acne. Indeed, people that can't produce or respond to growth hormones – such as those suffering from Laron syndrome, a disease that results in stunted growth – don't develop acne either [140]. But, as is the theme of this book, the causes for this disease are more complicated than this.

This additional twist comes from one observation made by researchers while studying men that are deficient in another class of hormones, one that promotes sex organ growth as opposed to systematic growth.

It was found that men who are deficient in sex hormones don't develop acne either, regardless of how much IGF-1 or other acne signals they receive. Remember that such hormones are secreted during puberty and cause gender-specific organs to grow to maturity. In the case of men, these hormones fall in the *androgens* group and drive testicle development, hair growth, and muscle development. As it happens, this class of hormones is also involved with skin health, making it the last major puzzle piece in our understanding of acne.

A time of maturing

Men that are deficient in androgens have normal reproductive organs specific to their sex, but they develop secondary sex characteristics that are more particular to women. For example, such men can have penises but go on to grow breasts during puberty. This dissonance is caused by a disagreement between the biological sex encoded in the DNA and how the body responds to sex hormones while growing up. It's a rare disorder, usually caused by insensitivity to androgens or the inability to convert testosterone into more potent androgens.

This disease is treatable, albeit somewhat tricky. It sometimes involves changing children's gender identity to match how they feel and how they respond to hormonal therapies. As you can imagine, changing your gender halfway through your childhood would be overwhelmingly confusing, which is why these adjustments need to be made with extreme care and consideration. Androgen deficiency is trickier to treat from a psychological perspective rather than physically.

But, if we ignore these aspects for now, one curious side effect of this disease is that people who are insensitive to androgens also do not develop acne [462]. Researchers found that people who can't produce or don't respond to androgens have a complete lack of sebum, even after going through puberty. More so, males who undergo hormone replacement therapy to reestablish secondary characteristics specific to their sex do develop acne and have normal sebum levels. This observation has led some researchers to speculate that acne depends on sex hormones, and that growth hormones are not enough to explain the explosion in acne cases we see during puberty.

In the early years of our life, the differences between boys and girls are much less proncunced than at maturity. Although we are born with organs specific to our sex, they are not fully functional until much later in our life. Sex organs fully develop around the age of

12 to 14 for girls and 12 to 16 for boys. Males experience growth in testis and penis size, while females experience menstruation and breast development. Some changes happen equally for boys and girls, such as the growth of pubic and armpit hair.

These changes are also governed by hormones secreted either by the brain directly or by organs specific to each sex. The sex differentiation signal starts from the brain through a hormone common to both men and women. It then travels through the bloodstream to organs specific to each sex (such as the testicles for men and ovaries for women). After the ovaries and testicles pick up this signal, more granular hormones are secreted by these organs that promote either male or female features.

The hormones that stimulate male organ development are called *androgens,* while the hormones that promote female development are called *estrogens.* Androgens are responsible for a wide range of male-related changes, including increased muscle mass, penis growth, broadening of the shoulders, voice deepening, etc. Similarly, estrogens trigger breast development, maturation of the vagina and uterus, and support ovarian functions in females.

Although androgens and estrogens are generally regarded as opposing forces, both are present in males and females but in different amounts. For example, androgen levels spike during puberty for young boys and girls. However, females experience lower overall levels of androgens, about one-twelfth the quantity compared to males [463]. These hormones are beneficial in women as well, as they are essential precursors to estrogens, supporting healthy female organ differentiation. Similarly, estrogens are also produced in males and play a crucial role in cognitive development and cardiovascular health [464]. Although androgens and estrogens are considered sex-specific hormones, both genders have a use for them.

We've already hinted a few times in this book that androgens are an essential factor in acne formation. This function comes as the result of androgen's role in har growth and maturation. This class of hormones triggers the local thickening of hair in some regions of the body (e.g., groin, armpits) [465] and, with this growth, sebum secretion [466].

In a way, androgens are responsible for healthy hair growth once we reach adulthood. In the absence of androgens, neither hairs nor sebum-producing cells mature fully. Although the SREBP transcription factors are the master regulators of all human lipids, androgens are the ones that control sebum production. Without androgens, you don't have sebum nor acne, no matter how much you activate SREBPs and other transcription factors.

As sebum is the main driving force behind acne, this makes androgens the necessary precursor for pimple growth. It doesn't matter if you're stressed, if you're eating junk food, or drinking loads of milk. As long as you don't have androgens, then you don't develop acne either. All the other transcription factors we've discussed so far are secondary to androgens. Overactivation of mTOR, FoxOs, or SREBPs doesn't affect our skin if these male sex hormones are not present.

You might be wondering why androgens, which are considered primarily male sex hormones, can affect women as well? The answer to this is quite simple: not all androgens are equally potent, and some organs can convert relatively inert forms of these hormones into more powerful versions. As it happens, the skin is one such organ that possesses specialized enzymes that can convert one form of androgen to another. We've mentioned this mechanism several times in this book when discussing the ability of some food items to influence this conversion process.

The precursors of androgens are much more balanced between men and women. *Dehydroepiandrosterone sulfate* (DHEA-S) is a weak androgen whose levels surpass testosterone by a factor of 100 to 500, even in men [467]. Levels of DHEA-S are approximately 40% lower in women than in men and gradually decline as we age, but still present in significantly higher quantities than classic androgens, such as testosterone [468].

For the most part, DHEA-S on its own is harmless with regards to acne, even acting as a suppressor of pimples in some scenarios. DHEA-S competes with other, more powerful androgens for the same receptors, thus blocking more potent hormones from working correctly. If hormone levels are just right, DHEA-S can hog androgen receptors, rendering them inert, thus decreasing their sebum-producing effect. DHEA-S really comes into play when it's converted into more powerful androgens in skin cells.

DHEA-S undergoes an entire chain of transformations before it can seriously stimulate androgen receptors and sebum secretion. It's first converted into intermediate hormones, such as *dehydroepiandrosterone (DHEA) and then* androstenedione. These intermediate hormones have some androgenic effects but very minor. From here, the hormones are further refined into *testosterone*, which is considered the primary male sex hormone, circulating in large quantities in males, but less so in females (males have, on average, eight times higher circulating testosterone levels compared to women) [469].

Testosterone is often used as a supplement by athletes to enhance performance by strengthening bones and increasing muscle mass. However, even though testosterone is the most common and utilized androgen, it's definitely not the most powerful. That spot is taken by the *dihydrotestosterone* (DHT) hormone, which is ten times more powerful than testosterone [318]. DHT can be produced from testosterone using the specialized enzymes that are present in our skin.

The entire chain of hormone transformation, from inert androgens to the most potent ones, looks something like this:

DHEA-S → DHEA → Androstenedione → Testosterone → DHT

Because DHEA-S can be converted to more powerful androgens, it likely plays a more important role in acne development than other androgens. It's true that women who have abnormally high levels of androgens (such as those suffering from *polycystic ovary syndrome)* are more prone to developing acne [318], but this wouldn't explain all acne cases in women. Instead, the comparable acne incidence rate between women and men can be explained by similar levels of androgen precursors that can be converted into testosterone and DHT by the skin without affecting secondary sex characteristics.

In one study, researchers found that DHEA-S levels were over twice as high in people with acne compared to clear-skin individuals [470]. This difference was observed both in women and in men. Considering that DHEA-S can be converted into testosterone and DHT directly in the skin, it makes sense to see this difference.

People prone to acne have higher circulating levels of these androgen precursors, stimulating the skin to produce more sebum, thus increasing the odds of pimples forming. As this hormone abnormality is found both in women and in men, gender doesn't play a role in androgen-driven acne. Both sexes can have atypical quantities of inert male sex hormones without developing male-specific sex organs.

In another similar study done only on young girls, it was found that blood levels of DHEA-S were a strong predictor of acne later in life. The scientists monitored adolescent girls from the firth grade up until three years after the first menstruation. The researchers found that girls who had elevated DHEA-S levels early in life had a higher chance of developing acne in adolescence (Figure 29 - DHEA-S versus acne lesions) [471].

These observations support the idea that acne is not a primary disease but more of a manifestation of other underlying problems in hormonal levels or diet imbalances. What's striking about this research is that these elevated DHEA-S levels were found several years before the first pimples appeared, indicating that these young girls suffered from undiagnosed hormone imbalances for most of their life. High levels of DHEA-S can cause other health issues besides affecting our skin, including irregular menstrual cycles, hair loss, fertility problems, and excessive body and facial hair [472].

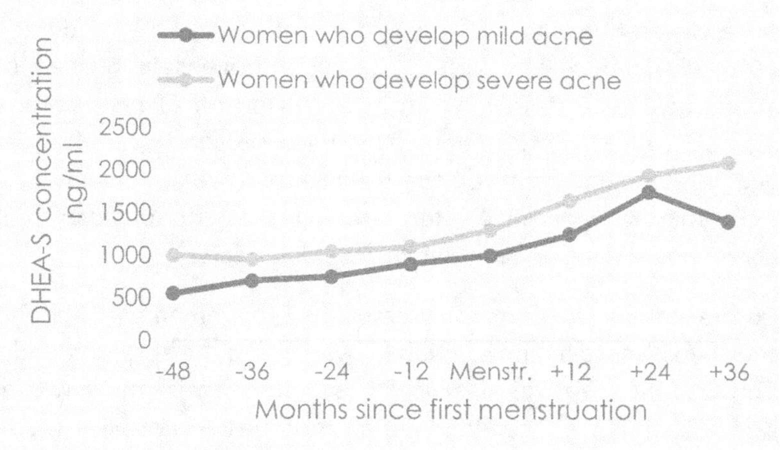

Figure 29 - DHEA-S versus acne lesions

Besides DHEA-S, young girls with acne also have elevated levels of the DHEA hormone, which is another weak androgen that can be converted into more powerful hormones through specialized enzymes [473]. It seems that acne, although dependant on male sex hormones, can also appear in people that are not "manly". DHEA-S and DHEA can be converted into acne promoters directly in the skin, leaving the secondary sex characteristics unaffected. However, although invisible, these hormones can cause other health problems if present in high enough quantities.

In a way, acne is a blessing for those that have it early on, as it shows the sufferers that they have internal imbalances that can create problems later in life and that it's a good idea to get tested for these hormones.

One advantage women have over men regarding androgen-driven acne is that they can use treatments that block or dull androgen receptors. Unfortunately, this is not a viable option for men, as a lack of androgens can have more severe health consequences for this gender, including non-functional sex organs, brittle bones, and a loss of muscle mass [474].

Women who elect to undergo hormonal therapy to treat acne have several options at their disposal: block the androgen receptors, reduce the production of androgens in ovaries or adrenal glands, or prevent the local conversion of testosterone into DHT. All of these options have been proven to be effective against acne, and all have been used as treatments in women for more than 30 years [475]. But, although these options can treat acne, they also come with significant side effects.

Contraceptives are commonly prescribed to women with acne as they block androgen production in ovaries and the adrenal glands. Certain contraceptives also block the androgen enzyme activity in skin cells, thus preventing the synthesis of the DHT hormone [475]. Yet, besides the obvious loss of fertility, contraceptives also increase the risk of developing complications in the arterial system, breast cancer, and myocardial infarction [475].

These adverse reactions were mostly seen in early contraceptives that had the side effect of increasing concentrations of estrogen and progestin in the blood. However, even with modern versions of these medications, it's still not advised to prescribe contraceptives to women with a generally higher risk of heart and circulatory problems.

There are safer ways to dull androgen receptors and prevent DHT production, and we've briefly touched on this subject during the

Alcohol chapter. In that chapter, we've mentioned that this conversion process is influenced by ethanols, as they activate the enzyme that transforms testosterone into DHT. But ethanol is not the only substance that affects this process.

Although all skin cells possess this ability of androgen conversion, we don't get thick hairs everywhere on our body. Instead, this enzyme activity happens in certain specialized places, such as the face or scalp [476]. This means that there must be other factors that affect localized hair growth and sebum production.

Although there is some genetic component to this process (in that some skin cells are genetically programmed to respond to androgens more than others), as we've seen throughout this book, genes are not immutable, and we can influence their behavior. The acne we get during puberty is not inescapable and is not entirely separate from the acne we get during adulthood.

To understand how and why, we first have to take a short refresher on all the major concepts learned throughout this book to see where androgens fit in the bigger picture. Once we do this, we can have a holistic view of this debilitating disease, to finally understand why our body goes out of balance and what we can do to restore it to optimal health.

A short refresher

In the introductory chapter of this book, we looked at the basic mechanisms through which pimples form. There, we saw that acne is primarily an inside-out disease, where clogs form within small chambers that are present throughout our skin. Through small sacks at the base of these chambers, our skin secretes an oily substance (named sebum) that lubricates our hairs and provides a protective layer against bacteria and other pathogens.

This oily substance usually travels from the base of skin pores, up the hair shaft, and then out onto the outer skin. However, if the mixture is too thick, it can create blockages, preventing the sebum's normal flow. If a clog is formed, pores will continue to build pressure as more and more sebum is produced. Once this pressure is high enough, the skin will rupture, spewing the accumulated sebum deeper within our skin. If this mixture also contains bacteria, it will trigger an inflammation response from our immune system, leading to pimples.

This mechanism of forming pimples applies to the most common acne version. However, throughout this book, we've learned that there are other forms of this disease. Acne can develop even without pore blockages if the skin is exposed to irritants that trigger an inflammation response. One such irritant is oxidized squalene, created when sebum is exposed to potent oxidation agents, commonly found in air pollutants or tobacco smoke. Similarly, we've also seen that excessive rubbing or prolonged pressure can also cause a different type of acne, named acne mechanica. There are many forms of this disease, but because classic acne is the most common one, we'll continue the discussion only for this variant.

For pimples to form, one or more of the following conditions must be met:

Sebum and flow composition are abnormal. Acne is primarily a sebum-driven disease, whereby pore plugs are created from sebum mixed with dead skin cells. A precondition of acne is to have thick and sticky sebum or sebum that is produced in large quantities. Androgens, high-glycemic foods, animal-derived proteins, and stress have been found to change either the flow rate or composition of sebum.

Skin cells die off at an abnormal rate. If skin cells die very quickly and in large quantities, the resulting junk will combine with sebum to form an even more viscous mixture. This process was found to be controlled by mTOR, as it drives cell reproduction and death. In turn, mTOR is influenced by foods with a high glycemic index, animal proteins, and growth hormones.

The immune system is overly active. Once skin pores become clogged, an overly-sensitive immune system can trigger inflammation easily, leading to more pimples or cystic acne.

Chocolate was the first item that we've found to put the immune system into overdrive, but general oxidative stress can also strain skin cells. Having few antioxidant agents circulating in our body will lead to a build-up of reactive oxidative species in the skin, thus promoting inflammation.

Bacterial growth on the skin is abnormal. The immune system will be more sensitive if exposed to sebum that contains higher quantities of bacteria. We've seen that excessive face scrubbing causes the migration of bacteria into skin pores, as that is the only place left with sebum. Once situated in skin pores, bacteria can quickly multiply, as they do not require oxygen for growth and reproduction. One other factor that causes excessive bacterial growth is the change in the composition of the sebum itself. If sebum is thicker, it will stick to the skin much better, creating a thin film over our skin that plants bacteria and helps it multiply freely.

At a cellular level, all these processes are governed by genes encoded in our DNA. This fact has lead to some speculation that acne is primarily a genetic disease, where some people are simply born with a predisposition to developing pimples later in life. However, throughout this book, we've seen that this is not necessarily true. For better or worse, genes can be molded and shaped through what we eat, how we interact with the environment, and our behavior.

On its own, a gene cannot influence the human body, as it's only information stored in our internal harddrive. Only after genes are converted into fully functioning proteins do we begin to feel their effect. This conversion process can be manipulated, essentially allowing us to turn on and off some genes. There are many ways to influence the production of proteins, but one method involves managing so-called gene transcription factors. They are specialized proteins that can either enhance or suppress the synthesis of genes.

For acne, we've seen that there are three key transcription factors that influence our susceptibility to this disease. SREBPs influence lipid production and, with it, sebum secretion. High SREBP activity leads to a higher sebum production with varying compositions, leading to an increased risk of pimples. Similarly, mTOR is a collection of multiple transcription factors that govern cell growth and division. These transcription factors oversee SREBPs, but they also manage other cellular processes that can exacerbate acne, including cell division, cell death, and inflammation. Lastly, FoxOs act as rheostats of SREBPs and mTOR, ensuring cell survival to the detriment of other non-essential cellular processes. FoxOs deactivate both SREBPs and mTOR, thus reducing the risk of acne.

The interplay between FoxOs, mTOR, and SREBP is the nucleus that shapes our understanding of how acne is formed and how to treat it. Each one of these transcription factors was found to influence the odds of developing acne in some way, either by directly controlling acne-promoting processes or by affecting each other. However, in this last chapter, we've seen that acne has another potent antagonist in the form of male sex hormones, also called androgens.

These hormones are secreted in abundance during puberty to stimulate the maturation of sex organs. Androgens are considered male sex hormones, as they support the development of male-specific organs and secondary features. Despite this, women also have an abundance of certain androgens, albeit versions that don't do much on their own. These hormones are inert, but they can be converted into more powerful varieties using specialized enzymes. Our skin possesses all such enzymes needed to convert androgens into potent forms, which is why it is more sensitive to the hormonal spike we have during puberty.

Androgens are the main drivers of sebum production and hair growth. They're the reason why our hair thickens and darkens in some areas of our bodies when we go through puberty. This is true for both women and men. Because the skin can convert weak androgens into more powerful versions, these hormones affect the skin of all sexes equally. Although the darkening of hair happens in different places in women and men, this change is still driven by male sex hormones. The same is true for sebum production.

Once we go through puberty, sebum production increases in all sexes equally, a process that is regulated by androgens. Because of this, some have called acne an androgen-dependant disease because you can't have pimples without these hormones stimulating sebum production. It was found that people that don't produce or don't respond to androgens don't develop acne either [477] [478]. This effect was found both in people who have rare genetic conditions that result in an inability to respond to sex hormones and in people who have lost the organs that produce androgens (e.g., castrated men).

Knowing this, one might assume that, to treat acne, we would have to fight on two fronts: mediate the three key transcription factors (mTOR, FoxOs, and SREBPs) and suppress androgen sensitivity. But, this is not necessarily true. The two paths we have to fight acne intersect more often than might appear.

Sebum production is expensive for the body. Throughout our life, it is estimated that we secrete up to 500Kg of sebum [479], which is more than six times as much as the average weight of a human being. Producing this much sebum consumes precious reserves of fat and other nutrients. Thus, it only makes sense to make sebum if we are eating enough, to not take away nutrients from critical systems that keep us alive. Ultimately, sebum is not essential to a person's survival, and when times are tough, our body can switch off these metabolic processes to conserve fat deposits.

This is why sebum production is mediated by transcription factors that sense our body's nutritional state and decide the appropriate levels of sebum to produce to keep us healthy. We've learned about one such transcription factor in the *Dairy* chapter. There, we saw that FoxOs are considered the master regulators of survival that can override many expensive bodily processes, including sebum-producing signals. When times are tough, they take over to ensure we make it to the next meal. Although comparably few Westerners are at risk of starvation, our bodies have not had enough time to adapt to the modern diet, hence why survival mechanisms still affect our health even today.

Sebum production is stimulated by many signals that can travel throughout our bodies. Most of this book was spent exploring growth hormones as a trigger of sebum, and we've seen that FoxOs can effectively cut this antenna in the sebum-producing glands. As it turns out, FoxOs also mediate the androgen signal that causes excessive sebum production, making this transcription factor the center point of our fight against this disease

The final link in our story is the same factor we've been coming back to, time and time again, one that differentiates nations with a high rate of acne from those in which this disease is non-existent. The reason why we have more acne cases during puberty is not because of some biological clock we can't escape, but because we have self-destructive habits that have become synonymous with modern civilizations. The connection between acne and puberty is, of course, our diet.

The final puzzle piece

For acne to form, skin cells must receive two signals: a growth signal, usually from the IGF-1 hormone; and a sex hormone signal. The first controls a multitude of transcription factors that give rise to acne, while the second controls sebum production itself. Although both messages are transmitted using hormones that circulate throughout our body, the most potent androgens are produced only locally in the skin. Particularly, DHT is the strongest hormone in this class. It is not present in our blood in any significant quantities, and it must be produced locally by our skin from testosterone (or other inert sex hormones) through special enzymes.

This simplistic view helps us understand why acne forms during puberty, as both hormones spike during this period. Growth hormones are produced to help our bodies grow and maturate into fully functioning adults, while sex hormones are secreted to accentuate the differences between biological males and females. Yet, this picture is not complete. It makes it seem like growth and sex hormones have very little in common, leading us to believe that we have to fight on two fronts to get rid of acne. In reality, however, they are more linked than might appear.

Many factors influence the enzyme activity that converts testosterone into DHT. Throughout this book, we've mentioned alcohol and stress as potential factors that dial up this enzyme activity, but recent evidence suggests that growth hormones can change this behavior as well.

When scientists took samples of skin cells and applied IGF-1 to them, they noticed that the enzyme activity that produces DHT increased significantly. After 4 hours since administering IGF-1, enzyme activity was seven times higher compared to normal [480]. When the researchers added substances that neutralize the IGF-1 hormone, the enzyme activity went back to normal, and DHT was no longer produced. Interestingly, this effect was not seen if the scientists introduced insulin instead of IGF-1 to the skin cells, even though both hormones can act as growth signals in some scenarios. It seems like this enzyme is affected only by IGF-1 and not by other similar hormones.

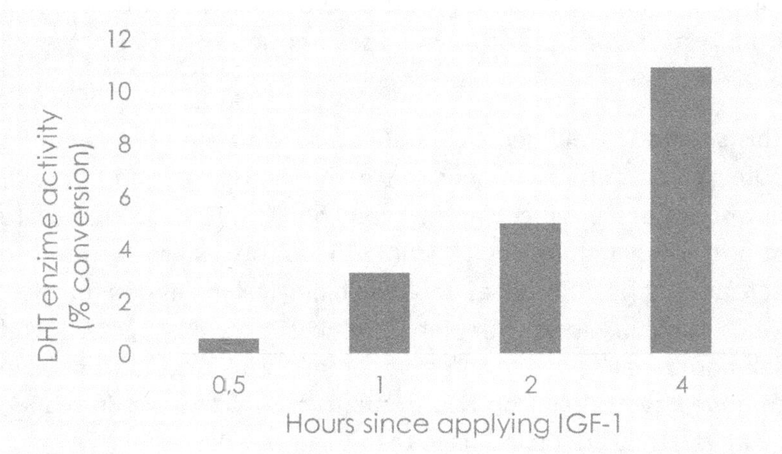

Figure 30 - IGF-1 influence over androgen conversion

IGF-1 doesn't affect only the production of more powerful androgens but also changes how sensitive the androgen receptors themselves are. Several in-vitro tests have shown that activation of androgen receptors is dependant on FoxO1 inhibition. If FoxO1 is present inside the nucleus, it blocks the activation of androgen receptors even if high quantities of androgens are present in the cell [481]. Inversely, if FoxO1 is forced out of the nucleus (for example, by some of the factors that we've mentioned throughout this book, including IGF-1), then this cancels its suppressive abilities, allowing androgen receptors to function correctly.

Researchers also found that FoxO1 prevents androgen receptors from being activated by signals other than androgens, such as some pro-inflammatory proteins [481]. Because of this, and because FoxO1 mediates most androgen antennas, this transcription factor is proving to be a central rheostat in androgen sensitivity as we l.

This interaction between FoxO1 and androgens was discovered while researching ways to prevent prostate cancer, as this disease also depends upon androgen activity [482]. This goes to show, once again, that acne is not really a primary disease in itself but is instead a manifestation of a severe imbalance in our bodies. If we treat only the superficial symptoms, we don't treat the underlying imbalances that can eventually lead to more severe health problems, including prostate cancer. Certain studies have even shown that men with acne early in life have a significantly increased risk of prostate cancer later in life [483].

The interplay between growth hormones and androgens explains why IGF-1 can be so damaging to our skin. On the one hand, IGF-1 stimulates the production of potent androgens by interfering with specialized enzymes in the skin. On the other hand, IGF-1 also prevents the protective effects of FoxO1 by forcing it out of the nucleus. On top of this, we've previously that IGF-1 also directly stimulates some transcription factors that can cause acne.

Interestingly, evidence suggests that a feedback loop between androgen receptors and IGF-1 receptors can develop, which amplifies this effect further. It was found that IGF-1 receptors are more sensitive when androgen receptors are activated [484]. Growth hormones make androgen receptors more likely to turn on, which in turn cause growth receptors to be more sensitive, and so on in an infinite circle.

This magnifying effect of IGF-1 explains why some people experience acne during puberty while others don't and why acne can persist well into adulthood for some. Although androgen levels are not significantly affected by our diet, sex hormones – and IGF-1 in particular – are. The spike in hormones that we get from eating certain foods is superimposed with hormones that are typically secreted during early childhood, to explode androgen sensitivity and the transcription factors that give rise to acne.

For healthy individuals, both androgens and sex hormones spike during puberty. This is usually a beneficial change, as it helps us grow and transform ourselves into healthy adults. However, this is valid only up to a certain point. IGF-1 spikes much higher in acne patients during puberty and is present for longer than normal, putting critical transcription factors and androgens into overdrive. This leads to pimples and other associated diseases.

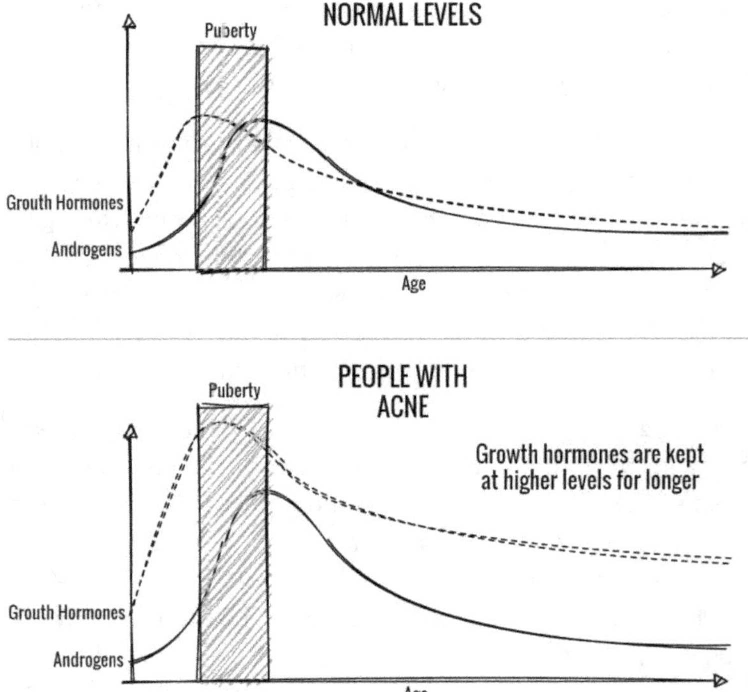

Figure 31 - Link between growth hormones and androgens

We're already discussed one major food group which conspires to keep IGF-1 levels artificially high, namely milk. The first connections between milk and acne were made as early as 1885 [485], but, since then, this link was strengthened through numerous studies that find that people who regularly drink milk or consume milk-derived products are at significant risk of developing acne [486]. This fact should come as no surprise, now that we know how devastating IGF-1 can be for our skin.

Milk is an exceptional food item, which has evolved to help frail newborns survive the first few months of their life. It's packed with growth hormones and proteins, needed to sustain life in its infancy when we are the most vulnerable. Because it's so protein-dense, athletes regularly consume concentrated dairy products to improve physical performance [139]. This might seem like it's a good thing, but putting anything into overdrive for extended periods will only do more harm than good in the long run.

It is well established that regular milk consumption increases serum levels of IGF-1 more than any other dietary food source [486]. Not only does it cause the body to produce more IGF-1 by interacting with the liver, but due to the nature of how the Dairy Industry operates, milk itself contains high amounts of growth and sex hormones. Cows must be kept pregnant to ensure milk production is consistent. As you can imagine, cows will only produce milk if there's a newborn calf that needs to be fed. For this reason, the majority of the milk we consume today comes from pregnant cows that are genetically engineered to produce more milk for longer [487].

To help support pregnancy and ensure normal fetal development, the adrenal glands of pregnant cows secrete copious amounts of the DHEA hormone. If you remember, this hormone can be converted to potent androgens in the skin through special enzymes, thus increasing sebum production in humans. Milk from pregnant cows contains 1.2 times more DHEA, 3.4 times more androstenedione, and 1.3 times more testosterone than non-pregnant cows [488]. Androgens can survive pasteurization [488] and digestion to be absorbed in the bloodstream [489]. Once in your body, these androgens that we get from milk will act identically to the human equivalent, instructing our skin to produce more sebum.

Although milk is likely the most dangerous food group in relation to acne, it shouldn't take the full blame. After all, the same studies that show that the risk of getting acne increases with milk consumption also show that people who never drink milk still get pimples (albeit at a lower rate) [490]. Milk alone is not enough to explain why we get acne.

As we've seen throughout this book, other food items, besides milk, also exacerbate acne. These foods are typical for Western diets and are consumed in much higher quantities in nations with high acne rates. One of the first food items that we've learned in this book and which poses a threat to our skin is meat and animal protein.

Animals that have a plant-based diet are able to accumulate all essential amino acids in their meat. Thus, animal tissue is a complete source of amino acids, which is why it is considered a superior source of nutrients. We would still get all essential amino acids even without eating meat, as long as we follow a diverse plant-based diet (similar to how the animals themselves eat). However, because it's easier just to eat these concentrated forms of proteins, athletes still only consume predominantly animal sources of protein. Despite meat's popularity, recent evidence suggests that it might be better to do the exact opposite to convention, as plant-based protein was found to support athletic performance better than animal protein [491] [492]. Even so, animal-based protein sources — such as meat, eggs, and dairy products — are consistently eaten in large quantities in Western nations due to their supposed health benefits.

Concerning acne, it is well known that animal protein is a potent stimulator of transcription factors that promote pimples. In the first few chapters, we've established that mTOR is one transcription factor that drives cell reproduction, inflammation, and sebum production, thus affecting several pathways that increase the risk of getting pimples.

mTOR is highly sensitive to animal protein, as it contains antennas that detect how well we are fed and if we are getting sufficient nutrients to sustain body growth. The amino acids from meat can easily activate these antennas. Yet, not all amino acids and proteins are equally dangerous – some protein sources activate mTOR more than others. In particular, leucine and arginine have been shown to have the highest influence over mTOR [493]. Leucine is found most abundantly in milk, more than any other source of animal protein; while arginine is found in copious amounts in certain meats, like turkey or beef [494].

Besides the interaction with mTOR, meat is now also thought to interplay with androgens and normal pubertal growth. It was found that children that consume high amounts of meat have higher androgens levels during puberty [495]. This imbalance in hormonal levels causes puberty to kick in earlier for these children, alongside all the bodily changes that are associated with this transitional phase [496]. These abnormalities can potentially aggravate acne as well, as we now know that androgens primarily drive this disease.

As with IGF-1, it seems that animal proteins interact with more than one factor that can cause acne, putting the body in a higher state of imbalance than what we initially thought. Meat promotes pimples by interfering with the normal functioning of the mTOR transcription factor while also increasing androgen sensitivity.

Another food group thought to cause pimples are high glycemic foods, usually eaten through refined carbohydrates. These, too, seem to cause complex changes to our bodies that make us more prone to breaking out.

Sugars and carbohydrates increase insulin levels (a hormone used by cells to absorb the energy stored in food). In turn, insulin stimulates mTOR to produce more dead skin cells, enhance inflammation, and increase sebum production. Additionally, insulin also forces FoxO1 out of the nucleus, preventing it from stopping the activation of androgen receptors. In this state, even tiny amounts of androgens can activate these receptors [497], thus causing even more sebum production. If these carb-driven changes are amplified by also eating meats and dairy products, our skin has no chance of defending itself against acne.

As you can see, our diet has a profound effect on the health of our skin. Taken one by one, each one of these food groups – milk, meat, and sugars – was found to interact with some components that make us more prone to breaking out. But, when taken whole, we now see that a diet based primarily on these foods leads to ramifications that are much more complex and much more damaging than what might seem.

Our body is not a collection of isolated pipes and components. Everything connects and interacts, such that one imbalance in our body can lead to faults in other places as well. It's hard for us to explain what all these interactions are, and we're far from understanding how everything connects, but the message is clear: the human body is more than the sum of its parts.

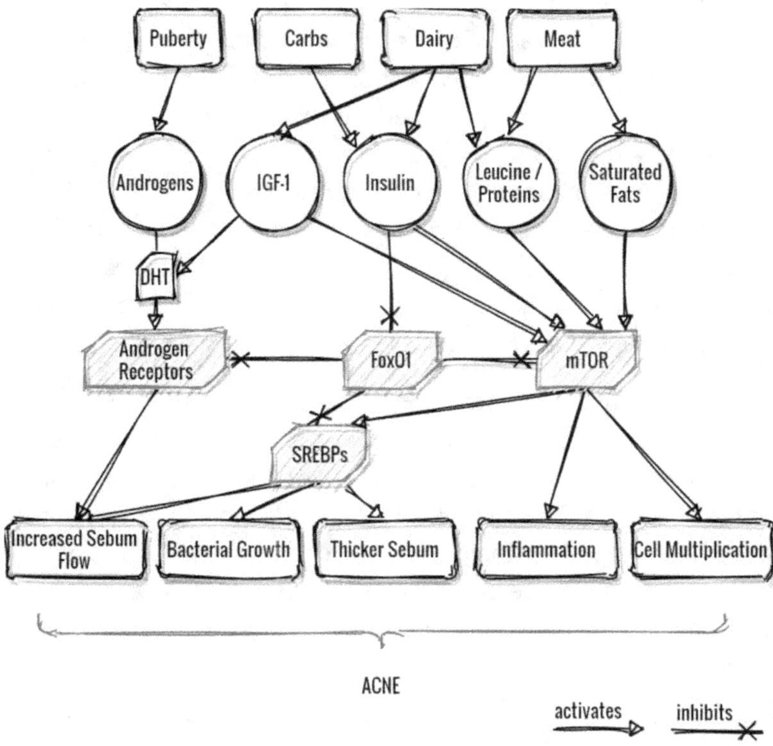

Figure 32 - Link between growth hormones and androgens

Modern humans have existed as a species for approximately 260,000 to 350,000 years [498]. Agriculture was first developed 11,500 years ago [499], while the first animals were domesticated even later, at around 10,000 before the current era [500]. Our species, as we know it today, evolved long before we discovered how to eat excessive carbohydrates (from cultivated grains), proteins (from meat sources), and hormones (from dairy products).

For 96% of the time our species existed, we only ate foraged plants and wild game. For 99.97% of our existence, we did not have a single hamburger [501]. The modern Western diet – rich in meat, fats, and carbs – has existed for only a few decades and was made possible with the advent of refrigeration and fast-food chains. This drastic change in diet in such a short period has not left humans enough time to evolve coping mechanisms for these new nutrients sources. Western diet puts our cells in a state of overdrive by supplying an abundance of sugars, hormones, and saturated fats. This promotes excessive sebum, cell death, inflammation, and bacterial growth, which eventually leads to acne. The Western diet also suppresses the ability of human cells to deal with stressful events, rendering useless our defense systems against acne.

As more and more countries continue to westernize, borrowing not only social but also culinary trends, acne incidence rates will continue to rise. This is evident from the recent explosion of acne cases in developing regions like Africa, the Middle East, and South-East Asia. If we persist in vehiculating common myths that acne is primarily caused by personal hygiene or genetic factors that we have no control over, this disease will continue to become more common.

The truth is that diet plays a much more important role in the health of our skin. Being conscious of this fact is paramount in our fight against this debilitating disease, one which creates not only long-lasting disfiguring scars but also emotional trauma, leading to a decreased quality of life and economic impact. Medication alone won't save us from this disease. We need to advance our understanding of what really causes this illness and how to recover from the systematic weakness that put us in this frail state.

Acne is not merely a skin-deep disease, as all the imbalances that lead to pimples were also found to promote other, more severe illnesses. A state of permanent mTOR activation has been linked to obesity, neurodegenerative diseases, and even cancer [502]. High androgen activity is associated with an increased risk of developing prostate cancer later in life [482]. Suppression of FoxO1 is correlated with a general higher mortality rate [503]. Similarly,

SREBPs are involved in the development of fatty liver disease, hepatitis, and hepatic cancer [504].

In a way, acne can be considered a blessing, as it allows us to see that something serious is wrong within our body, giving us a chance to improve our health before it becomes too late. When we have the flu, we don't take medication to treat just the sneezing. Instead, we treat the underlying infection that put us in that state. Once we recognize that acne is not merely a superficial disease that can be treated by over-the-counter creams and lotions, we will be able to regain our health and our life.

CHAPTER SUMMARY

- For pimples to form, our skin requires two broad signals: a growth signal that affects acne-promoting transcription factors (SREBPs, mTOR, FoxO1) and an androgen signal that increases sebum production.

- During puberty, growth and androgen hormones spike at roughly the same time. When both are at their peak, we have the highest chance of developing pimples.

- Hormone levels can be changed through what we eat. Foods such as dairy and meat promote the production of growth hormones. Milk also contains precursors to androgens, essentially providing both acne signals.

- Certain growth hormones (such as IGF-1) promote the conversion of inert androgens to more potent versions. For these reasons, foods that increase blood IGF-1 levels are especially hazardous to our skin, as they can activate both nutrient and growth antennas all at once.

- The Western diet is the perfect blend that drives all these internal changes that give rise to acne. This diet is high in animal protein, which stimulates various transcription factors that promote acne. It is also high in saturated and trans-fats that alters the chemical composition of sebum to make it thicker and more prone to blockages. Similarly, Westerners also eat foods that change normal hormonal levels, affecting sensors that are present in sebum-producing cells.

- Acne is not an inescapable disease brought by Mother Nature. Instead, it is created by humans and shaped by what we eat.

EASY REFERENCE LIST

What to avoid

- Dairy products (and especially whey protein)
- High-glycemic foods (carbohydrates, sugar)
- Leucine-rich animal products (milk, meat, eggs)
- Cocoa-based products (chocolate)
- Saturated fats
- Excess alcohol
- Sunflower seeds
- Pollution
- Stress

What to get more of

- Fruits, veggies, and berries (especially Barberries)
- Green tea
- Foods rich in unsaturated fats (vegetable oils, nuts)
- Tea tree oil (applied on acne-prone skin)

BOOK SUMMARY

- Acne is a common disease, especially among adolescents, but only in some nations. Notably, regions that we consider "Western" have the highest incidence of acne.

- This difference in acne prevalence can be explained by factors that are unique to Western nations, including their diet and lifestyle choices.

- Our skin is extremely sensitive to what we eat and has antennas that listen to changes in blood glucose levels, protein concentrations, and some hormones. When these nutrients are consumed in excess, it gives rise to sebum flow increases and compositional changes, a heightened sensitivity to inflammation, and excessive bacterial growth. All these changes can make us more prone to breaking out.

- Our skin is also sensitive to damage from the environment, such as highly reactive chemicals resulting from air pollution or smoking.

- The Western lifestyle contains all stimulants that make us more prone to breaking out: it provides excess nutrients (particularly from milk, meat, and refined carbs), and it exposes us to highly reactive gases that irritate our skin (from air pollution and smoking).

- There is no evidence to suggest that hygiene has any major role in acne development.

- Acne is really a sign that a severe imbalance is happening in our bodies, such as excessive production of growth and sex hormones, an improper balance between saturated and unsaturated fats, and heightened activity in gene regulators. These imbalances can give rise to more serious conditions down the line if left untreated, including cancers, neurodegenerative diseases, and diabetes.

- Dietary changes can take up to 12 weeks to show improvements to our skin. Be patient and consistent if you're planning to alter your lifestyle to improve your health.

REFERENCES

[1]   P. Loren Cordain, M. P. Staffan Lindeberg, P. Magdalena Hurtado and e. al, "Acne Vulgaris - A Disease of Western Civilization".

[2]   G. D. Kellett SC, "The psychological and emotional impact of acne and the effect of treatment with isotretinoi".

[3]   B. G. F. S. e. a. Rapp DA, "Anger and acne: implications for quality of life, patient satisfaction and clinical care".

[4]   "Global Acne Drugs Market Report 2020 featuring Major Players - Allergan, Galderma, Valeant Pharma, Teva Pharmaceutical and Johnson & Johnson," [Online]. Available: https://www.reportlinker.com/p05251482/Global-Acne-Market-Report-for.html.

[5]   K. V. K. Y. F. J K Tan, "Beliefs and perceptions of patients with acne".

[6]   "Global Acne Market Report for 2016-2026," 2017.

[7]   https://www.drugwatch.com/accutane/lawsuits/.

[8]   K. A. P. P. C. H. Mills OH Jr, "Comparing 2.5%, 5%, and 10% benzoyl peroxide on inflammatory acne vulgaris.".

[9]   T. K. Makoto Kawashima Toshitaka Nagare, "Open-label, randomized, multicenter, phase III study to evaluate the safety and efficacy of benzoyl peroxide gel in long-term use in patients with acne vulgaris: A secondary publication".

[10]   W. J. B. N. Rademaker M1, "Isotretinoin 5 mg daily for low-grade adult acne vulgaris--a placebo-controlled, randomized double-blind study.".

[11]   K. O. C. M. B. M. A. J. Opel D, "Not every patient needs a triglyceride check, but all can get pancreatitis: a systematic review and clinical characterization of isotretinoin-associated pancreatitis.".

[12]   https://vizhub.healthdata.org/gbd-compare/.

REFERENCES

[13]   https://web.archive.org/web/20131207163839/http://www.staffanlindeberg.com/TheKitavaStudy.html.

[14]   P. N.-E. A. T. B. V. B. S. S. LINDEBERG, "Cardiovascular risk factors in a Melanesian population apparently free from stroke and ischaemic heart disease : the Kitava study".

[15]   M. D. K.-M. S. Q. G. M. a. C. L. O. P. Cheryl D. Fryar, "Mean Body Weight, Height, Waist Circumference, and Body Mass Index Among Adults: United States,1999–2000 Through 2015–2016".

[16]   "Age relations of cardiovascular risk factors in a traditional Melanesian society: the Kitava Study".

[17]   A. H. S. H. &. F. T. Chew, "Systematic review of the epidemiology of acne vulgaris".

[18]   G. V. CHCunliffe, "WJ The familial risk of adult acne: a comparison between first-degree relatives of affected and unaffected individuals.".

[19]   D. M. S. Mathieu Laplante, "mTOR signaling in growth control and disease".

[20]   T. A. F. A. Humyra Tabasum, "The Historic Panorama of Acne Vulgaris".

[21]   https://web.archive.org/web/20130415053448/http://www.articledashboard.com/Article/History-Of-Acne/2912672.

[22]   B. M. P. R. M. a. K. N. Ariel Eva Eber, "Acne treatment in antiquity: can approaches from the past berelevant in the future?".

[23]   G. Tilles, "Acne Pathogenesis: History of Concepts".

[24]   T. Arif, "Salicylic acid as a peeling agent: a comprehensive review".

[25]   H. Y. J. X. L. L. G. L. H. S. F. P. Haibo Liu, "Evidence-based topical treatments (azelaic acid, salicylic acid, nicotinamide, sulfur, zinc, and fruit acid) for acne: an abridged version of a Cochrane systematic review".

[26]   M. O. E. C. A. M. Mauro Picardo, "Sebaceous gland lipids".

[27]   P. R. a. B. G. H. Nicole M. Avena, "Evidence for sugar addiction: Behavioral and neurochemical effects of intermittent, excessive sugar intake".

[28]   A. Z. V. R. C. E. W. N. D. V. G.-J. W. Clara R Freeman, "Impact of sugar on the body, brain, and behavior".

[29]   "World Health Organization. Guideline: Sugars intake for adults and children.".

[30]   "IDF EUROPE POSITION ON ADDED SUGAR," 2016.

[31]   K. J. Clifton PM, "A systematic review of the effect of dietary saturated and polyunsaturated fat on heart disease.".

[32]   K. C. T. S. T. S. A. A. I. H. M. S. F. K. Y. Y. O. Y. A. Y. S. H. Horikawa C and J. D. C. S. Group., "Meat intake and incidence of cardiovascular disease in Japanese patients with type 2 diabetes: analysis of the Japan Diabetes Complications Study (JDCS)".

[33]   W. S. M. D. Micha R, "Red and processed meat consumption and risk of incident coronary heart disease, stroke, and diabetes mellitus: a systematic review and meta-analysi".

[34]   S. A. B. (. T. C. CrowePhD, "Low-carbohydrate diets: what are the potential short- and long-term health implications?".

[35]   P. I. R. A. J. K. Y.-C. L. Jørgen Jensen, "The Role of Skeletal Muscle Glycogen Breakdown for Regulation of Insulin Sensitivity by Exercise".

[36]   S. B. H. M. H. S. A. J. P. R. M. Y. S. Dympna Gallagher, "Healthy percentage body fat ranges: an approach for developing guidelines based on body mass index".

[37]   K. F.-P. J. C. B.-M. Fiona S. Atkinson, "International Tables of Glycemic Index and Glycemic Load Values: 2008".

[38]   Z. J. L. J. Z. S. X. Y. H. Y. J. D. C. L. Z. X. S. J. K. Y. Z. W. C. M. C. X. S. M. Huang X, "Daily Intake of Soft Drinks and Moderate-to-Severe Acne Vulgaris in Chinese Adolescents".

[39]   M. L. D. P. H. E. M. L. C. M. D. D. M. E. B. M. Amanda Suggs MD, "An Acne Survey from the World's Largest Annual Gathering of Twins".

REFERENCES

[40] B. İ. S. H. K. S. K. K. Y. M. A. D. Ö. S. K. G. Ç. A. B. S. T. E. D. M. U. T. G. S. A. A. F. A. A. B. Ç. E. E. Ö. T. Karadağ AS1, "The effect of personal, familial, and environmental characteristics on acne vulgaris: a prospective, multicenter, case controlled study from Turkey.".

[41] M. R. K. R. Nguyen QG, "Diet and acne: an exploratory survey study of patient beliefs.".

[42] S. N. Veith WB, "The association of acne vulgaris with diet.".

[43] N. J. M. A. B. H. M. G. A. V. Robyn N Smith, "A low-glycemic-load diet improves symptoms in acne vulgaris patients: a randomized controlled trial".

[44] D. ZD, "The effect of a daily facial cleanser for normal to oily skin on the skin barrier of subjects with acne".

[45] J. Y. Y. J. S. H. J. Y. J. M. S. P. D. H. S. Hyuck Hoon Kwon, "Clinical and Histological Effect of a Low Glycaemic Load Diet in Treatment of Acne Vulgaris in Korean Patients: A Randomized, Controlled Trial".

[46] S. J. R. W. W. K. Burris J, "A Low Glycemic Index and Glycemic Load Diet Decreases Insulin-like Growth Factor-1 among Adults with Moderate and Severe Acne: A Short-Duration, 2-Week Randomized Controlled Trial".

[47] M. H. 2. New York, "McGraw-Hill Encyclopedia of Science and Technology'.

[48] J. G. C. P. Renaud Dentin, "Carbohydrate responsive element binding protein (ChREBP)and sterol regulatory element binding protein-1c (SREBP-1c) two key regulators of glucose metabolism and lipid synthesis in liver".

[49] R. S. Hitoshi Shimano, "SREBP-regulated lipid metabolism: convergent physiology — divergent pathophysiology".

[50] K. G. G. A. C. D. T. Terry M. Smith, "IGF-1 induces SREBP-1 expression and lipogenesis in SEB-1 sebocytes via activation of the Phosphoinositide 3-kinase (PI3-K)/Akt pathway".

[51] https://pubchem.ncbi.nlm.nih.gov/compound/Oleic-acid#section=Decomposition.

[52]   https://pubchem.ncbi.nlm.nih.gov/compound/squalene#section=Stability-Shelf-Life.

[53]   B. C. Melnik, "Western diet-induced imbalances of FoxO1 and mTORC1 signallingpromote the sebofollicular inflammasomopathy acne vulgaris".

[54]   C. W. H. K. Gribbon EM, "Interaction of Propionibac-terium acnes with skin lipids in vitro".

[55]   I. T. H. K. I. S. D. M. Katsuta Y, "Function of oleic acid on epidermal barrier and calcium influx into keratinocytes is associated with N-methyl D-aspartate-type glutamate receptors.".

[56]   "Vegetarianism in America," *vegetariantimes.*

[57]   H. Ritchie, "How much of the world's land would we need in order to feed the global population with the average diet of a given country?".

[58]   M. K. M. C. L. C. N. H. H. R. J. H. W. A. L. Christiane A. Opitz, "Damped elastic recoil of the titin spring in myofibrils of human myocardium".

[59]   E. R. M. Katherine Hoy, M. John C. Clemens and M. R. Alanna Moshfegh, "What We Eat in America".

[60]   https://www.health.harvard.edu/nutrition/when-it-comes-to-protein-how-much-is-too-much.

[61]   D. J. a. E. H.George Mandel, "Effect of dietary protein level on aflatoxin Bj actions in the liver ofweanling rats".

[62]   T. C. C. B S Appleton, "Inhibition of aflatoxin-initiated preneoplastic liver lesions by low dietary protein".

[63]   T. C. Campbell, "Dietary protein, growth factors, and cancer".

[64]   B. Seto, "Rapamycin and mTOR: a serendipitous discovery and implications for breast cancer".

[65]   S. M. Douros J, "New antitumor substances of natural origin.".

[66]   M. V. Blagosklonny, "Rapamycin for longevity: opinion article".

REFERENCES

[67]   S. R. S. Z. N. J. A. C. F. K. N. N. W. J. F. K. C. C. P. M. J. M. F. E. M. R. Harrison DE, "Rapamycin fed late in life extends lifespan in genetically heterogeneous mice.".

[68]   J. M. T. F. K. C. S. J. J. A. F. L. P. Ivana Bjedov, "Mechanisms of Life Span Extension by Rapamycin in the Fruit Fly Drosophila melanogaster".

[69]   S. G. K. a. J. B. Jing Li, "Rapalogs and mTOR inhibitors as anti-aging therapeutics. The Journal of clinical investigation.".

[70]   S. F. S. K. B. K. T. J. M. F. Zachary A Knight, "A critical role for mTORC1 in erythropoiesis and anemia".

[71]   L. S. B. S. G. T. K. D. Vander Haar E, "Insulin signalling to mTOR mediated by the Akt/PKB substrate PRAS40.".

[72]   X.-h. Y. Xiu-zhi Li, "Sensors for the mTORC1 pathway regulated by amino acids".

[73]   L. S. Yun CW, "The Roles of Autophagy in Cancer.".

[74]   W. B. W. Y. Huang F, "Role of autophagy in tumorigenesis, metastasis, targeted therapy and drug resistance of hepatocellular carcinoma.".

[75]   S. M. S. S. Fujikake N, "Association Between Autophagy and Neurodegenerative Diseases.".

[76]   P. C. T. N. Metaxakis A, "Autophagy in Age-Associated Neurodegeneration.".

[77]   B. H. D. C. P. D. Z. M. R. M. S. I. E.-H. N. K. F. Pleet ML, "Autophagy, EVs, and Infections: A Perfect Question for a Perfect Time.".

[78]   V. S. S. E. S. S. K. D. Sharma V, "Selective Autophagy and Xenophagy in Infection and Disease.".

[79]   T. Y. Shuhei Nakamura, "Autophagy and Longevity".

[80]   N. a. S. N. Hay, "Upstream and downstream of mTOR".

[81]   C. R. S. B. G. M. C. M. W. S. L. J. R. G. Y.-L. C. A. S. Thomas Porstmann, "SREBP Activity Is Regulated by mTORC1 and Contributes to Akt-Dependent Cell Growth".

[82]   B. Melnik, "Dietary intervention in acne".

[83]   V. D. D. F. O. E. Pierdominici M, "mTOR signaling and metabolic regulation of T cells: new potential therapeutic targets in autoimmune diseases.".

[84]   D. G. M. C. C. W. P. J. Zheng Y, "Anergic T cells are metabolically anergic".

[85]   H. D. R. S. T. K. C W. Jeremy AH, "Inflammatory events are involved in acne lesion initiation".

[86]   K. J. T. L. B. M. B. S. T. S. Young CN, "Reactive oxygen species in tumor necrosis factor-alpha-activated primary human keratinocytes: implications for psoriasis and inflammatory skin disease.".

[87]   C. B. Thomas Jonathan Stewart, "Hormonal and dietary factors in acne vulgaris versus controls".

[88]   S. T., "Acne and Whey Protein Supplementation among Bodybuilders".

[89]   https://nutritiondata.self.com/facts/sausages-and-luncheon-meats/1390/2.

[90]   https://nutritiondata.self.com/facts/vegetables-and-vegetable-products/2761/2.

[91]   T. J. Madhulika B Gupta, "Novel roles of mechanistic target of rapamycin signaling in regulating fetal growth".

[92]   S. T. G. M. K. W. S. G. B. R. Z. E. S. A. L. J. G. D. Bodine SC, "Akt/mTOR pathway is a crucial regulator of skeletal muscle hypertrophy and can prevent muscle atrophy in vivo.".

[93]   "'There's something terribly wrong': Why more Americans are dying in middle age," [Online]. Available: https://www.advisory.com/daily-briefing/2019/12/02/middle-age-death.

[94]   G. X. K. I. W. M. W. M. S. M. A. A. Hughes KC, "Intake of dairy foods and risk of Parkinson disease.".

[95]   R. G. P. H. M. K. L. L. N. J. W. L. T. C. Abbott RD1, "Midlife milk consumption and substantia nigra neuron density at death.".

[96]   B. J. M. L. S. M. E. M. H. N. W. A. J. J. A. O. F. K. A. S. Downer M, "Dairy intake in relation to prostate cancer survival.".

REFERENCES

[97]   M. J. K. S. W. K. E. R. S. B. D. K. Chia JSJ, "A1 beta-casein milk protein and other environmental pre-disposing factors for type 1 diabetes.".

[98]   W.-T. D. G.-J. L. Jing-Zhang Wang, "Limit the uptake of milk by young people: A method to prevent the occurrence of heart failure".

[99]   B. H. S. C. H. G. K. S. I. K. D. H. S. M. N. D. B. S. S. S. L. Bechthold A, "Food groups and risk of coronary heart disease, stroke and heart failure: A systematic review and dose-response meta-analysis of prospective studies".

[100]   T. T. Engel S, "Butter increased total and LDL cholesterol compared with olive oil but resulted in higher HDL cholesterol compared with a habitual diet.".

[101]   C. A. C. M. Nestel PJ, "Dairy fat in cheese raises LDL cholesterol less than that in butter in mildly hypercholesterolaemic subjects.".

[102]   L. W. T. V. B. S. G. G. G. A. R. I. Bolland MJ, "Calcium intake and risk of fracture: systematic review.".

[103]   L. M. V. A. N. B. E. C. Bergholdt HKM, "Lactase persistence, milk intake, hip fracture and bone mineral density: a study of 97 811 Danish individuals and a meta-analysis".

[104]   R. J. K. Robert G. Cumming, "Case-Control Study of Risk Factors for Hip Fractures in the Elderly".

[105]   O. ES., "The effects of dietary protein insuf-ficiency and excess on skeletal hea th.".

[106]   "https://www.usda.gov/media/blog/2017/09/26/back-basics-all-about-myplate-food-groups".

[107]   *https://www.reportbuyer.com/product/2262903/Global-Dairy-Industry---The-Milky-Way.html.*

[108]   "International Monetary Fund - World Economic Outlook Database".

[109]   M. G. MD, *The Saturated Fat Studies: Buttering Up the Public.*

[110]   J. A. A. L. J. e. a. E. J. E. Guo, "Milk and dairy consumption and risk of cardiovascular diseases and all-cause mortality: dose–response meta-analysis of prospective cohort studies," [Online].

[111]   R. Collier, "Dairy research: "Real" science or marketing?".

[112]   E. B. F. D. J. H. M. Ulvestad, "Acne and dairy products in adolescence: results from a Norwegian longitudinal study," [Online].

[113]   C. A. D. C. S. F. W. H. H. G. A. W. C. M. D. Adebamowo, *Milk consumption and acne in adolescent girls.*

[114]   B. H. M. I. J. G. K. J. E. C. Juhl CR, "Dairy Intake and Acne Vulgaris: A Systematic Review".

[115]   V. S. S. J. G. C. P. V. P. V. P. C. H. N. B. A. C. N. F. N. B. A. J. M. L. Y. W. S. B. Y. Chanet A, "Supplementing Breakfast with a Vitamin D and Leucine-Enriched Whey Protein Medical Nutrition Drink Enhances Postprandial Muscle Protein Synthesis and Muscle Mass in Healthy Older Men.".

[116]   K. C. T. G. T. J. M. R. G. F. M. S. B. F. M. L. H. P. S. Rondanelli M, "Whey protein, amino acids, and vitamin D supplementation with physical activity increases fat-free mass and strength, functionality, and quality of life and decreases inflammation in sarcopenic elderly.".

[117]   G. C. C. Y. G. D. L. J. Fekete ÁA, "Whey protein lowers blood pressure and improves endothelial function and lipid biomarkers in adults with prehypertension and mild hypertension: results from the chronic Whey2Go randomized controlled trial.".

[118]   A. S. S. M. M. W. E. M. D. West DWD, "Whey Protein Supplementation Enhances Whole Body Protein Metabolism and Performance Recovery after Resistance Exercise: A Double-Blind Crossover Study".

[119]   N. A. N. A. S. H. K. G. I. P. G. C. M. B. E. B. H. R. T. Hamarsland H, "Native whey protein with high levels of leucine results in similar post-exercise muscular anabolic responses as regular whey protein: a randomized controlled trial".

[120]   H. S. G. S. M. P. Chungchunlam SM, "Effect of whey protein and a free amino acid mixture simulating whey protein on measures of satiety in normal-weight women".

[121]   L. F. L. Y. T. Y. K. X. F. Z. A. T. W. M. H. Y. W. G. Y. Y. Duan Y, "The role of leucine and its metabolites in protein and energy metabolism.".

[122]   https://www.myfooddata.com/articles/high-leucine-foods.php.

REFERENCES

[123]   M. Appleby, "The Amino Acid Profile of an Apple".

[124]   G. M. C. F. F. d. S. P. T. J. F. S. F. Thaís de Carvalho Pontes, "Incidence of acne vulgaris in young adult users of protein-calorie supplements in the city of João Pessoa".

[125]   N. G. K. S. A. a. B. S. K. Vandana Dhaka, "Trans fats—sources, health risks and alternative approach - A review".

[126]   T. Y. K. S. e. a. Yasuda M, "Fatty acids are novel nutrient factors to regulate mTORC1 lysosomal localization and apoptosis in podocytes".

[127]   M. Y. Y. S. U. M. J. S. H. Y. S. C. D. H. S. Jae Yoon JUNG, "The influence of dietary patterns on acne vulgarisin Koreans".

[128]   M. R. C. Jennifer Burris, M. M. William Rietkerk and P. R. F. Kathleen Woolf, "Relationships of Self-Reported Dietary Factors andPerceived Acne Severity in a Cohort of New YorkYoung Adults".

[129]   https://www.nutritionvalue.org.

[130]   https://fdc.nal.usda.gov/.

[131]   M. J. P. B. M. K. Zuzana Havlicekova, "Beta-palmitate − a natural component of human milk in supplemental milk formulas".

[132]   A. B. B. M. B. D. T.-G. M. T. D. T. A. L. E. A. B. J. P. C. P. L. B. Brassard D, "Saturated Fats from Butter but Not from Cheese Increase HDL-Mediated Cholesterol Efflux Capacity from J774 Macrophages in Men and Women with Abdominal Obesity".

[133]   L. H. A. Daphna K Dror, "Overview of Nutrients in Human Milk".

[134]   B. C. Melnik, "Excessive Leucine-mTORC1-Signalling of Cow Milk-Based Infant Formula: The Missing Link to Understand Early Childhood Obesity".

[135]   S. D. D. F. F. A. W. W. H. M. Adebamowo CA, "High school dietary dairy intake and teenage acne.".

[136]   M. BC, "Evidence for acne-promoting effects of milk and other insulinotropic dairy products.".

[137]   M. B., "Milk consumption: aggravating factor of acne and promoter of chronic diseases of Western societies.".

[138]   D. L. R. S. O. K. G. H. T. A. O. A. C.-C. F. B.-R. M. B. H. L. P. L. J. N. G. T. A. T. D. K. V. S. S. P. D. P. S. T. R. S. C. Norat T, "Diet, serum insulin-like growth factor-I and IGF-binding protein-3 in European women".

[139]   G. D. P. M. Rich-Edwards JW, "Milk consumption and the prepubertal somatotropic axis.".

[140]   J. S. S. G. Melnik BC, "Over-stimulation of insulin/IGF-1 signaling by western diet may promote diseases of civilization: lessons learnt from laron syndrome".

[141]   P.-Y. W. T. K. K. H. A. S. Li-Qiang Qina, "Estrogen: one of the risk factors in milk".

[142]   B. K. K. K. H. G. H. Kindahla, "Endocrine changes in late bovine pregnancy withspecial emphasis on fetal well-being".

[143]   W. W. T. R. .. F. A. S. M. C. L. Crystal J. Kirby, "Effects of Growth Hormone and Pregnancy on Expression of Growth HormoneReceptor, Insulin-Like Growth Factor-I, and Insulin-Like Growth Factor BindingProtein-2 and -3 Genes in Bovine Uterus, Ovary, and Oviduct".

[144]   https://www.cancer.org/cancer/cancer-causes/recombinant-bovine-growth-hormone.html.

[145]   R. K. K. S. Venkateswarlu Sunkesula, "Review: Milk and Milk Products, Insulin-like Growth Factor-1 and Cancer".

[146]   M. R. KLASS, "A METHOD FOR THE ISOLATION OF LONGEVITY MUTANTS IN THE NEMATODE CAENORHABDITIS ELEGANS AND INITIAL RESULTS".

[147]   T. E. J. D. B. Friedman, "A Mutation in the Age-1 Gene in Caenorhabditis Elegans Lengthens Life and Reduces Hermaphrodite Fertility".

[148]   https://www.livescience.com/52843-acorn-worm-genome-sequencing.html.

[149]   L. P. Maria E. Giannakou, "Role of insulin-like signalling in Drosophila lifespan".

[150]   K. B. K. C. Bluher M, "Extended longevity in mice lacking the insulin receptor in adipose tissue.".

REFERENCES

[151]   G. J. L. W. L. Rute Martins, "Long live FOXO: unraveling the role of FOXO proteins in aging and longevity".

[152]   S.-M. J. P. T. B. V. N. D. I. T. Y. P. a. N. H. Chia-Chen Chen, "FoxOs inhibit mTORC1 and activate Akt by inducing theexpression of Sestrin3 and Rictor".

[153]   X. W. M. T. N. L. H. B. Allison Birnbaum, "Age-Dependent Changes in Transcription Factor FOXO Targeting in Female Drosophila".

[154]   M. M. J. M. S. N. L. P. Tettweiler G, "Starvation and oxidative stress resistance in Drosophila are mediated through the eIF4E-binding protein, d4E-BP.".

[155]   A. D. S. O. M. B. Y. D. Agamia NF, "Skin expression of mammalian target of rapamycin and forkhead box transcription factor O1, and serum insulin-like growth factor-1 in patients with acne vulgaris and their relationship with diet".

[156]   J. J. B. H. S. C C. Z. M. P. P. Wesley J. Harrison, "Expression of Lipogenic Factors Galectin-12, Resistin,SREBP-1, and SCD in Human Sebaceous Glands andCultured Sebocytes".

[157]   A. Q. Y. K. X. K. J. L. R. W. X. O. J. Z. Y. C. F. F. Xiaojun Liu, "FoxO1 represses LXRa-mediated transcriptional activity of SREBP-1c promoterin HepG2 cells".

[158]   L. G. B. M. Z. I. A. A. C. P. I. T. S. J. H. M. Becker T, "FOXO-dependent regulation of innate immune homeostasis.".

[159]   M. S. Lorna Moll, "The Role of Insulin and Insulin-Like Growth Factor-1/FoxO-Mediated Transcription for the Pathogenesis of Obesity-Associated Dementia".

[160]   B. C. Melnik, "Linking diet to acne metabolomics, inflammation, and comedogenesis: an update".

[161]   https://tools.myfooddata.com/nutrition-facts/172475/100g/1.

[162]   https://tools.myfooddata.com/nutrition-facts/171269/100g/1.

[163]   c. a. G. J. W. D. K. L. a. C. J. M. a. P. J. G. Layne E Norton, "Leucine content of dietary proteins is a determinant of postprandial skeletal muscle protein synthesis in adult rats".

[164]   N. M. A. A. N. G. Erica M. Schulte, "Which Foods May Be Addictive? The Roles of Processing, Fat Content, and Glycemic Load".

[165]   "The Global Chocolate Market size is expected to reach $171.6 billion by 2026, rising at a market growth of 5.3% CAGR during the forecast period," [Online]. Available: https://www.globenewswire.com/news-release/2020/06/12/2047602/0/en/The-Global-Chocolate-Market-size-is-expected-to-reach-171-6-billion-by-2026-rising-at-a-market-growth-of-5-3-CAGR-during-the-forecast-period.html.

[166]   G. D. F. T. G. R. C. D. G. G. C. A. D. C. P. P. Maria Teresa Montagna, "Chocolate, "Food of the Gods": History, Science, and Human Health".

[167]   "The Sweet History of Chocolate," [Online]. Available: https://www.history.com/news/the-sweet-history-of-chocolate.

[168]   R. Latif, "Chocolate/cocoa and human health: a review".

[169]   L. Y. S. X. e. a. Ren Y, "Chocolate consumption and risk of cardiovascular diseases: a meta-analysis of prospective studies".

[170]   R. M. R. K. Quynh-Giao Nguyen, "Diet and acne: an exploratory survey study".

[171]   J. M. James E. Fulton, M. Gerd Plewig and M. P. and Albert M. Klingman, "Effects of Chocolate on Acne Vulgaris".

[172]   F. D. M. T. E. B. a. L. L. Jon A HalvorsenEmail author, "Is the association between acne and mental distress influenced by diet? Results from a cross-sectional population study among 3775 late adolescents in Oslo, Norway".

[173]   B. S. V. M. K. J. B. B. Caperton C, "Double-blind, Placebo-controlled Study Assessing the Effect of Chocolate Consumption in Subjects with a History of Acne Vulgaris.".

[174]   M. a. P. A. M. D. Saivaree Vongraviopap, "Dark chocolate exacerbates acne".

[175]   A. D. D. S. R. C. A. N. Panche, "Flavonoids: an overview".

[176]   C. M. Pérez-Cano FJ, "Flavonoids, Inflammation and Immune System.".

[177]   M. S. R. G. Spagnuolo C, "Anti-inflammatory effects of flavonoids in neurodegenerative disorders.".

REFERENCES

[178]   M. M. S. B. R. S. M. R. B. L. Goya L, "Effect of Cocoa and Its Flavonoids on Biomarkers of Inflammation: Studies of Cell Culture, Animals and Humans.".

[179]   K. D. A. A. David L. Katz, "Cocoa and Chocolate in Human Health and Disease".

[180]   S. A. J. M. J. T. J. L. J. G. M.-T. T. S. P. M. G. N. L. A. B. J. Stejara A. Netea, "Chocolate consumption modulates cytokine production in healthy individuals".

[181]   A.-M. H. a. U. W. Maike van Ohlen, "Herbivore Adaptations to Plant Cyanide Defenses".

[182]   D. M. S. C. M. J. S. J. Aleksandra Radanović, "Sunflower Genetics from Ancestors to Modern Hybrids—A Review".

[183]   J. Whelan, "Linoleic Acid".

[184]   J. K. .J. Goldberg, "A meta-analysis of the analgesic effects of omega-3 poly-unsaturated fatty acid supplementation for inflammatory joint pain".

[185]   L. AC., "Linoleic and linolenic acids and acne vulgaris".

[186]   H. R. K. S. W. K. M. S. S. S.-J. L. J. H. &. L. H.-S. Lee, "The efficacy and safety of gamma-linolenic acid for thetreatment of acne vulgaris".

[187]   K. H. H. J. Y. J. P. M. J. M. S. D. Jung JY, "Effect of dietary supplementation with omega-3 fatty acid and gamma-linolenic acid on acne vulgaris: a randomised, double-blind, controlled trial.".

[188]   Z. V. Chapkin RS, "Inability of skin enzyme preparations to biosynthesize arachidonic acid from linoleic acid.".

[189]   S. J. J.-C. L. M. E. Apostolos Pappas, "Sebum analysis of individuals with and without acne".

[190]   ,. B. a. P. LETAWE, "Digital image analysis of the effect of topically applied linoleic acid on acne microcomedones.".

[191]   R. L. Gallo, "Human Skin Is the Largest Epithelial Surface for Interaction with Microbes".

[192]   S.-B. H. M. M. Mohebbipour A, "Sunflower Seed and Acne Vulgaris.".

[193]   R.-F. S. M. M. E. Arshad Z, "The Sources of Essential Fatty Acids for Allergic and Cancer Patients; a Connection with Insight into Mammalian Target of Rapamycin: A Narrative Review".

[194]   S. D. B. E. e. a. Menon D, "Lipid sensing by mTOR complexes via de novo synthesis of phosphatidic acid".

[195]   B. S. S. L. B. J. A. W. P. T. M. S. K. R. B. R. G. K. Ornish D, "Can lifestyle changes reverse coronary heart disease? The Lifestyle Heart Trial".

[196]   S. S. L. W. Tuso P, "A plant-based diet, atherogenesis, and coronary artery disease prevention".

[197]   R. G. B. Kathleen E. Adair1, "Ameliorating Chronic Kidney Disease Using a Whole Food Plant-Based Diet".

[198]   H. F. D. C. J. G. A. L. Christina Osland Johannesen, "Effects of Plant-Based Diets on Outcomes Related to Glucose Metabolism: A Systematic Review".

[199]   I. M. H. B. B. C. Tuso PJ, "Nutritional Update for Physicians: Plant-Based Diets".

[200]   Y. P. H. Z. L. Q. T. X. H.-C. W. H.-D. C. C.-D. H. B Wei, "The epidemiology of adolescent acne in North East China".

[201]   C. S. C. F. B. A. C. C. M. M. P. A. B. V. P. E. C. M. F. A. C. E. I. V. N. L. Di Landro A and G. f. E. R. i. D. A. S. Group., "Adult female acne and associated risk factors: Results of a multicenter case-control study in Italy.".

[202]   T. VV., "GENETIC AND EPIGENETIC CAUSES OF OBESITY".

[203]   N. T. H. J. Nielsen LA., "The Impact of Familial Predisposition to Obesity and Cardiovascular Disease on Childhood Obesity".

[204]   F. J. B. L. Savage JS, "Parental Influence on Eating Behavior".

[205]   J. MD., "Reactive oxygen species and programmed cell death".

[206]   B. T. Y. Y. F. B. M. C. B. T. N. R. Tarique Hussain, "Oxidative Stress and Inflammation: What Polyphenols Can Do for Us?".

[207]   A. H. T. J. Diana B Holland, "The Role of Inflammation in the Pathogenesis of Acne and Acne Scarring".

REFERENCES

[208] M. Emil A. Tanghetti, "The Role of Inflammation in the Pathology of Acne".

[209] P. M. K. A. Mills OH, "Enhancement of comedogenic substances by ultraviolet radiation".

[210] M. GE, "Use of vitamin C in acne vulgaris".

[211] "Mangosteens Arrive, but Be Prepared to Pay," [Online]. Available: https://www.nytimes.com/2007/08/08/dining/08mang.html.

[212] I. P. N. S. M. H. D. Obolskiy, "Garcinia mangostana L.: a phytochemical and pharmacological review".

[213] N. C.-R. M. O.-I. J. P.-R. J. Pedraza-Chaverri, "ROS scavenging capacity and neuroprotective effect of α-mangostin against 3-nitropropionic acid in cerebellar granule neurons".

[214] Q. S. W. Z. B. S. J.J. Wang, "Anti-skin cancer properties of phenolic-rich extract from the pericarp of mangosteen (Garcinia mangostana Linn.)".

[215] B. S. W. K. R. M. A. K. H.A. Jung, "Antioxidant xanthones from the pericarp of Garcinia mangostana (Mangosteen)".

[216] L. Y. C. W. L G. Chen, "Anti-inflammatory activity of mangostins from Garcinia mangostana".

[217] S. S. V. S. N. W. G. Mullika Traidej Chomnawang, "Antimicrobial effects of Thai medicinal plants".

[218] "Exports of mangosteen from Thailand up 400% in the first six months," vol. Thailand Headlines.

[219] W. A. K. C. C. N. W. S. Pan-In P, "Depositing α-mangostin nanoparticles to sebaceous gland area for acne treatment".

[220] The divine farmer's materia medica : a translation of the Shen Nong Ben Cao Jing. Yang, Shouzhong.

[221] B. A. Cicero AF, Berberine and Its Role in Chronic Disease..

[222] L. P. T. M. S. A. Ortiz LM, Berberine, an epiphany against cancer..

[223]   M. Z. Q. S. K. R. A. C. M. U. Y. S. S. B. N. S. T. P. P. B. X. Ammad Ahmad Farooqi, "Regulation of Cell Signaling Pathways by Berberinein Different Cancers: Searching for Missing Pieces of an Incomplete Jig-Saw Puzzle for an Effective Cancer Therapy".

[224]   f. a. t. c. o. J.-C. t. h. m. o. t. l. o. s. g. Effect of some alkaloids, "Seki T, Morohashi M.".

[225]   R. F. Fouladi, "Aqueous Extract of Dried Fruit ofBerberisvulgaris L.in Acne vulgaris, a Clinical Trial".

[226]   G. G. D. J. G. M. R. M. Esselstyn CB Jr, "A way to reverse CAD?".

[227]   "The Actual Benefit of Diet vs. Drugs," [Online]. Available: https://nutritionfacts.org/video/the-actual-benefit-of-diet-vs-drugs/.

[228]   W. C. M. M. H. V. Worrapan Poomanee, "In-vitro investigation of anti-acne properties of Mangifera indica L. kernel extract".

[229]   B. G. R. P. D. W. E. H. K. R. B. N. H. Coenye T, "Eradication of Propionibacterium acnes biofilms by plant extracts and putative identification of icariin, resveratrol and salidroside as active compounds.".

[230]   A. N. A. A. Khan H, "Effects of Cream Containing Ficus carica L. Fruit Extract on Skin Parameters: In vivo Evaluation.".

[231]   S. P. D. J. C. K. K. T. H. S. K. J. F. S. Li Z, "Antimicrobial Activity of Pomegranate and Green Tea Extract on Propionibacterium Acnes, Propionibacterium Granulosum, Staphylococcus Aureus and Staphylococcus Epidermidis.".

[232]   A. J. K. A. L. E. K. J. M. Y. Lee HH, "Chemical composition and antimicrobial activity of the essential oil of apricot seed.".

[233]   D. M. B. M. O. S. Ilknur T, "Glycolic acid peels versus amino fruit acid peels for acne.".

[234]   "Benefits of Amino Fruit Acid for Acne & How to Use it," [Online]. Available: https://healthyy.net/acne/chemical-peels/amino-fruit-acid-use.

REFERENCES

[235]   O. Y. L. J. Z. M. Z. G. B. W. H. F. Wang X, "Fruit and vegetable consumption and mortality from all causes, cardiovascular disease, and cancer: systematic review and dose-response meta-analysis of prospective cohort studies".

[236]   C. W. M. K. C. E. W. W. E. A. Farvid MS, "Fruit and vegetable consumption in adolescence and early adulthood and risk of breast cancer: population based cohort study.".

[237]   W. M., "The Second World Cancer Research Fund/American Institute for Cancer Research Expert Report. Food, Nutrition, Physical Activity, and the Prevention of Cancer: A Global Perspective: Nutrition Society and BAPEN Medical Symposium on 'Nutrition supp".

[238]   I. F. M. J. H. F. W. W. v. D. R. S. Q. Muraki I, "Fruit consumption and risk of type 2 diabetes: results from three prospective longitudinal cohort studies.".

[239]   C. M. Lembo A, "Chronic constipation.".

[240]   *OECD.Stat,* https://stats.oecd.org/Index.aspx?DataSetCode=SHA.

[241]   "2019 Human Development Index Ranking," [Online]. Available: http://hdr.undp.org/en/content/2019-human-development-index-ranking.

[242]   "U.S. Life Expectancy 1950-2020," [Online]. Available: https://www.macrotrends.net/countries/USA/united-states/life-expectancy.

[243]   M. M. Howard K. Koh, M. M. Anand K. Parekh and M. M. John J. Park, "Confronting the Rise and Fall of US Life Expectancy," [Online].

[244]   P. A. W. D. L. X. D. K. F. O. K. S. D. A. E. S. M. W. W. H. F. Li Y, "Impact of Healthy Lifestyle Factors on Life Expectancies in the US Population.".

[245]   https://twitter.com/odavis_/status/793579307893395456?ref_src=t wsrc%5Etfw.

[246]   *Cost?, How Much Does an Ambulance Ride,* https://www.howmuchisit.org/ambulance-ride-cost/.

[247]   S. M. A. S. Chetty R, "heassociation between income and life expectancy inthe United States, 2001-2014.".

[248]   M. C. K. A. Totri CR, "Kids These Days: Urine as a Home Remedy for Acne Vulgaris?'.

[249]   A. C. T. T. Ages, "Sarah Marshall, Michael Magnes".

[250]   E. N. Johnson, "Traditional medicine for modern times: Facts and figures".

[251]   "Herbal Medicine Market Size and Forecast, By Product (Tablets & Capsules, Powders, Extracts), By Indication (Digestive Disorders, Respiratory Disorders, Blood Disorders), And Trend Analysis, 2014 - 2024".

[252]   https://pubmed.ncbi.nlm.nih.gov/?term=green+tea.

[253]   "https://pubmed.ncbi.nlm.nih.gov/?term=garlic," [Online].

[254]   A. Simonson, "Another War Fought Over Tea - The Opium Wars".

[255]   *History, Chinese Tea History Part I - Green Tea,* https://www.teavivre.com/info/green-tea-history.html.

[256]   "Tea Consumption Second Only to Packaged Water," [Online]. Available: https://worldteanews.com/tea-industry-news-and-features/tea-consumption-second-only-to-packaged-water.

[257]   B. C. D. J. Z. D. L. U. B. S. Mancini E, "Green tea effects on cognition, mood and human brain function: A systematic review.".

[258]   Y. H. T. N. K. Y. H. S. N. J. U. Y. S. Y. Ide K, "Effects of green tea consumption on cognitive dysfunction in an elderly population: a randomized placebo-controlled study.".

[259]   Z. F. C. P. Z. K. X. H. M. Q. W. X. Z. X. Guo Y, "Green tea and the risk of prostate cancer: A systematic review and meta-analysis.".

[260]   C. H. Z. L. L. G. Y. D. Z. Y. W. Y. L. X. W. X. S. Q. L. L. Y. D. Huang Y, "Association between green tea intake and risk of gastric cancer: a systematic review and dose-response meta-analysis of observational studies.".

[261]   N. S. K. Y. Y. H. M. A. I. K. N. Y. Unno K, "Ingestion of green tea with lowered caffeine improves sleep quality of the elderly via suppression of stress.".

REFERENCES

[262] N. S. K. Y. Y. H. M. A. I. K. N. Y. Unno K, "Reduced Stress and Improved Sleep Quality Caused by Green Tea Are Associated with a Reduced Caffeine Content.".

[263] G. S. M. P. I. M. N. Y. Ohishi T, "Anti-inflammatory Action of Green Tea.".

[264] L. C. C. J. H. C. Chen IJ, "Therapeutic effect of high-dose green tea extract on weight reduction: A randomized, double-blind, placebo-controlled clinical trial.".

[265] M. H. Khan N, "Tea Polyphenols in Promotion of Human Health".

[266] G. H.N., "Green tea composition, consumption, and polyphenol chemistry".

[267] F. A. M. S. N. A. H. M. Naghma Khan, "Targeting Multiple Signaling Pathways by Green Tea Polyphenol (–)-Epigallocatechin-3-Gallate".

[268] C. J. T. W. P. H. Z. L. C. R. T. P. L. L. Van Aller G.S., "Epigallocatechin gallate (EGCG), a major component of green tea, is a dual phosphoinositide-3-kinase/mTOR inhibitor.".

[269] K. H. M. S. T. D. S. D. Yoon J.Y., "Epigallocatechin-3-gallate improves acne in humans by modulating intracellular molecular targets and inhibiting P. Acnes. J. Investig. Dermatol.".

[270] "Cholesterol," [Online]. Available: https://www.britannica.com/science/cholesterol.

[271] W. C. Reygaert, "The antimicrobial possibilities of green tea".

[272] N. R. Jaclyn M. Forest, "Oral Aqueous Green Tea Extract and Acne Vulgaris: A Placebo-Controlled Study".

[273] P. D. B. R. Bassett IB, "A comparative study of tea-tree oil versus benzoylperoxide in the treatment of acne.".

[274] d.-b. p.-c. s. The efficacy of 5% topical tea tree oil gel in mild to moderate acne vulgaris: a randomized, "Bassett IB, Pannowitz DL, Barnetson RS.".

[275] N. A. A.-S. M. Sharquie KE, "Topical therapy of acne vulgaris using 2% tea lotion in comparison with 5% zinc sulphate solution.".

[276]   T. J. R. T. K. S. H. K. Malhi HK, "Tea tree oil gel for mild to moderate acne; a 12 week uncontrolled, open-label phase II pilot study.".

[277]   S. S. K. M. V. H. H. B. Deepak M. Kasote, "Significance of Antioxidant Potential of Plants and its Relevance to Therapeutic Applications".

[278]   "How many MAP are used world-wide?," [Online]. Available: http://www.fao.org/3/AA010E/AA010e02.htm.

[279]   M. Seki T, "Effect of some alkaloids, flavonoids and triterpenoids, contents of Japanese-Chinese traditional herbal medicines, on the lipogenesis of sebaceous glands".

[280]   B. K. T. M. R. P. M. Q. M. A. N. Akhtar, "Formulation and evaluation of antisebum secretion effects of sea buckthorn w/o emulsion".

[281]   H. Dobrev, "Clinical and instrumental study of the efficacy of a new sebum control cream".

[282]   K. S. S. Y. C. I. Nam C, "Anti-acne effects of Oriental herb extracts: a novel screening method to select anti-acne agents.".

[283]   A. L. E. G. P. S. Jain, "Anti-inflammatory effects of Erythromycin and Tetracycline on Propionibacterium. acnes induced production of chemotactic factors and reactive oxygen species by human neutrophils".

[284]   S. K. T. O. N. L. C. H. W.J. Yoon, "Abies koreana essential oil inhibits drug-resistant skin pathogen growth and LPS-induced inflammatory effects of murine macrophage".

[285]   H. J. J. C. Y. K. S. K. H. K. H. Lim, "Anti-inflammatory activity of the constituents of the roots of Aralia continentalis".

[286]   S. K. M. J. I. H. W. W. K.H. Kim, "Anti-inflammatory phenylpropanoid glycosides from Clerodendron trichotomum leaves".

[287]   R. E. J. G. A. B. A. R. H. G. R. Enk, "Differential effect of Rhizoma coptidis and its main alkaloid compound berberine on TNF-alpha induced NFkappaB translocation in human keratinocytes".

[288]   R. S. A. S. J. H. M. Sharma, "The potential use of Echinacea in acne: control of Propionibacterium acnes growth and inflammation".

REFERENCES

[289]   T. T. W. W. J. T. P. T. T.H. Tsai, "In vitro antimicrobial and anti-inflammatory effects of herbs against Propionibacterium acnes".

[290]   E. A. A. O. O. B. O. O. F. A. L.O. Orafidiya, "The effect of aloe vera gel on the anti-acne properties of the essential oil of Ocimum gratissimum Linn leaf — a preliminary clinical investigation".

[291]   J. L. E. J. Y. P. K. K. B. P. e. a. J. Park, "In vitro antibacterial and anti-inflammatory effects of honokiol and magnolol against Propionibacterium sp.".

[292]   S. T. S. Y. P. Panichayupakaranant, "Antibacterial, anti-inflammatory and anti-allergic activities of standardised omegranate rind extract".

[293]   S. J. S. K. J. C. K. H. d. I. L. S.S. Joo, "Anti-acne activity of Selaginella involvens extract and its non-antibiotic antimicrobial potential on Propionibacterium acnes".

[294]   N. A. B. K. H. K. T. S. T. Mahmood, "Outcomes of 3% green tea emulsion on skin sebum production in male volunteers".

[295]   M. F.-T. A. A. K. M. A. Hanieh Azimi, "A review of phytotherapy of acne vulgaris: Perspective of new pharmacological treatments".

[296]   A. O. D. O. C.O. Alebiosu, "A report of clinical trial conducted on Toto ointment and soap products".

[297]   J. A. C. P. W. S. P.J. Magin, "Topical and oral CAM in acne: a review of the empirical evidence and a consideration of its context".

[298]   A. J. A. S. F. I. S. Enshaieh, "The efficacy of 5% topical tea tree oil gel in mild to moderate acne vulgaris: a randomized, double-blind placebo-controlled study".

[299]   E. E. K.W. Martin, "Herbal medicines for treatment of bacterial infections: a review of controlled clinical trials".

[300]   V. S. B. S. K. G. Ravichandran, "Evaluation of efficacy and safety of Acne-N-Pimple cream in acne vulgaris".

[301]   H. Dobrev, "Clinical and instrumental study of the efficacy of a new sebum control cream".

[302]   "WHO Guidelines on Hand Hygiene in Health Care: First Global Patient Safety Challenge Clean Care Is Safer Care.".

[303]   J. Dingman, "How did we discover the first virus?".

[304]   S. Riedel, "Edward Jenner and the history of smallpox and vaccination".

[305]   D. B. Goldstein, "Effect of Alcohol on Cellular Membranes".

[306]   J. A. H. I. M. M. R. G. C. G. G. K. N. H. S. Manuela G. Neumana, "Ethanol signals for apoptosis in cultured skin cells".

[307]   K. B. M. S. L. D. Y. M. K. N. K. Y. L. E. R. Y. K. K. Suh DH, "A multicenter epidemiological study of acne vulgaris in Korea.".

[308]   V. S. G. H. S. A. Karciauskiene J, "The prevalence and risk factors of adolescent acne among schoolchildren in Lithuania: a cross-sectional study.".

[309]   D. a. U. T. a. D. R. a. D. C. Lynn, "The epidemiology of acne vulgaris in late adolescence".

[310]   J. S. S. G. Melnik BC, "Milk is not just food but most likely a genetic transfection system activating mTORC1 signaling for postnatal growth".

[311]   R. Y. A. A. B. K. Röjdmark S, "Insulin-like growth factor (IGF)-1 and IGF-binding protein-1 concentrations in serum of normal subjects after alcohol ingestion: evidence for decreased IGF-1 bioavailability.".

[312]   "Alcohol-related liver disease," [Online]. Available: https://www.nhs.uk/conditions/alcohol-related-liver-disease-arld/.

[313]   N. Chalasani, Z. Younossi, J. E. Lavine, M. Charlton, K. Cusi, M. Rinella, S. A. Harrison, E. M. Brunt and A. J. Sanyal, "The diagnosis and management of nonalcoholic fatty liver disease: Practice guidance from the American Association for the Study of Liver Diseases".

[314]   M. A. J. S. S. M. PETER E. POCHI, "SEBACEOUS GLAND RESPONSE IN MAN TO THE ADMINISTRATION".

[315]   H.-P. T. E. a. Yi-Chien Yang, "Female Gender and Acne Disease Are Jointly and Independently Associated with the Risk of Major Depression and Suicide: A National Population-Based Study".

[316]   W. J. Hay ID, "Clinical Endocrine Oncology.".

REFERENCES

[317]   G. G. G. A. L. S. S. C. R. P. R. M. C. S. L. J Vittek, "Effect of ethanol intake on cellular regulation of testosterone-5 alpha-reductase in rat oral tissues.".

[318]   M. DIANE THIBOUTOT, "Acne: Hormonal Concepts and Therapy".

[319]   E. C. Sarkola T, "Testosterone increases in men after a low dose of alcohol.".

[320]   E. C. Apter SJ, "The effect of alcohol on testosterone concentrations in alcohol-preferring and non-preferring rat lines".

[321]   B. v. d. Pahlen, "The Role of Alcohol and steroid hormones in human aggregssion".

[322]   C. f. D. C. a. Prevention, "Alcohol Use and Your Health," [Online]. Available: https://www.cdc.gov/alcohol/fact-sheets/alcohol-use.htm.

[323]   P. Anderson, "The impact of alcohol on health".

[324]   W. H. Organization, "Alcohol in the European Union".

[325]   "Global salt consumption to reach 335 million tons," [Online]. Available: https://www.foodexecutive.com/en/marketing/2096-global-salt-consumption-raises.html.

[326]   "Salt intake," [Online]. Available: https://www.who.int/data/gho/indicator-metadata-registry/imr-details/3082.

[327]   M. O. A. Z. M. D. M. A. H. M. R. A. H. M. D. K. M. D. I. S. M. H. S. A. P. M. A. S. M. P. M. A. El Darouti, "Salty and spicy food; are they involved in the pathogenesis of acne vulgaris?".

[328]   G. LE., "Salt restriction in acne vulgaris".

[329]   S. P. Suckling RJ, "The health impacts of dietary sodium and a low-salt diet.".

[330]   E. I. F. H. S. K. S. M. Philipson H, "Salt and fluid restriction is effective in patients with chronic heart failure.".

[331]   "Edema," [Online]. Available: https://www.mayoclinic.org/diseases-conditions/edema/symptoms-causes/syc-20366493.

[332]   B. V. K. L. B. a. A. B. K. M. M. Joanna Mimi Choi, "A Single-Blinded, Randomized, Controlled Clinical Trial Evaluating the Effect of Face Washing on Acne Vulgaris".

[333]   A. A. U. I. A. R. T. M. R. K. Haroon MZ, "Quality Of Life And Depression Among Young Patients Suffering From Acne.".

[334]   Y. Y. K. M. S. A. Bez Y, "High social phobia frequency and related disability in patients with acne vulgaris.".

[335]   M. S. Matsui, "Update on Diet and Acne".

[336]   M. Heather L. Brannon, "What Is Sebum and How Does Your Skin Produce It?".

[337]   J. H. Ovhal A, "A comparative study of sebum secretion rates and skin types in individuals with and without acne".

[338]   "Women are gravitating towards more natural ingredients, while also adding more products, and using them more frequently," [Online]. Available: https://www.npd.com/wps/portal/npd/us/news/press-releases/2017/for-nearly-half-of-us-women-using-facial-skincare-products-ingredients-determine-their-purchases/.

[339]   "Skin Care Products Market Worth $183.03 Billion By 2025 | CAGR: 4.4%," [Online]. Available: https://www.grandviewresearch.com/press-release/global-skin-care-products-market.

[340]   https://data.worldbank.org/indicator/NY.GDP.MKTP.CD?year_high_desc=true.

[341]   B. S. Del Rosso JQ, "The Role of Skin Care as an Integral Component in the Management of Acne Vulgaris: Part 2: Tolerability and Performance of a Designated Skin Care Regimen Using a Foam Wash and Moisturizer SPF 30 in Patients with Acne Vulgaris Undergoing Active Treatment.".

[342]   K. B. J.K.L. Tan, "A global perspective on the epidemiology of acne".

[343]   S. E. C. S. R. F. Karen E Huang, "The Duration of Acne Treatment".

[344]   P. P. K. M. S. K. G. A. M. a. R. G. T. Sharmila Sarkar, "Personality disorders and its association with anxiety and depression among patients of severe acne: A cross-sectional study from Eastern India".

REFERENCES

[345]   K. R. A. G. R. K. E. L. &. A. A. N. Florian Anzengruber, "Wide range of age of onset and low referral ratesto psychiatry in a large cohort of acne excoriée ata Swiss tertiary hospital".

[346]   L. M. K. E. A. M. D. L. R. T. S. Nancy J. Keuthen, "The prevalence of pathologic skin picking in US adults".

[347]   G. A. S. N. Gupta MA, "Psychological factors affecting self-excoriative behavior in women with mild-to-moderate facial acne vulgaris.".

[348]   M. E. A. K. G. M. F. N. J. S. M. MADHULIKA A. GUPTA, "PSYCHOSOMATIC STUDY OF SELF-EXCORIATIVEBEHAVIOR AMONG MALE ACNE PATIENTS:PRELIMINARY OBSERVATIONS".

[349]   K. Mills OH, "Acne mechanica".

[350]   "Ambient air pollution: Health impacts," [Online]. Available: https://www.who.int/airpollution/ambient/health-impacts/en/.

[351]   G. S. D. Isangedighi Asuquo Isangedighi, "Heavy Metals Contamination in Fish: Effects on Human Health".

[352]   K. D. W. MacNee, "Mechanism of lung injury caused by PM10 and ultrafine particles with special reference to COPD".

[353]   W. H. Organization, "Health effects of particulate matter," 2013.

[354]   S. C. P. A. C. F. C. C. M. E. Valacchi G, "Cutaneous responses to environmental stressors".

[355]   B. R. W. M. H. G. A. Z. H. B. S. M. S. E. W. G. D. K. N. M. X. W. F. P. E. K. S. M. T. A. R. F. d. H. K. K. T. E. M. P. P. Raaschou-Nielsen O, "Particulate matter air pollution components and risk for lung cancer.".

[356]   https://www.esa.int/Applications/Observing_the_Earth/Is_the_ozon e_layer_on_the_road_to_recovery.

[357]   "Rethinking the ozone problem in urban and regional air pollution".

[358]   K. J. Delimpasis, "Ozone and Color Removal".

[359]   H. A. V. M. G. P. a. M. F. d. M. Videla, "The Effect of Ozonated Cooling Water on the Corrosion Behavior of Stainless Steel, Titanium and Copper Allcys; Ozone Biocidal Action on Sessile and Planktonic Bacteri".

[360]   J. E. P. M. Zouboulis CC, "Acne is an inflammatory disease and alterations of sebum composition initiate acne lesions.".

[361]   G. o. o. s. i. h. c. m. f. v. o. exposure, "J. Cotovio, L. Onno, P. Justine, S. Lamure, P. Catroux".

[362]   D. M. W. L. S. K. G.-S. L. N. N. L. F. X. S. S. Jean Krutmann, "Pollution and acne: is there a link?".

[363]   L. O. P. J. S. L. P. C. J Cotovio, "Generation of Oxidative Stress in Human Cutaneous Models Following in Vitro Ozone Exposure".

[364]   S. S. D. MOYAL, "EFFECT OF AIR POLLUTION ON SEBUM RATE AND ACNE: HOW TO MANAGE ACNEIC SKIN IN A POLLUTED ENVIRONMENT".

[365]   W. Z. Y. H. L. Y. Z. Z. F. Z. Y. Z. L. Y. S. L. B. Y. Q. Y. P. R. C. B. H. D. C. O. d. L. S Nouveau-Richard, "Oily Skin: Specific Features in Chinese Women".

[366]   X. P. A. V. Q. G. X. W. Q. W. S. S. D. M. T. S. J. K. Wei Liu, "A Time-Series Study of the Effect of Air Pollution on Outpatient Visits for Acne Vulgaris in Beijing".

[367]   W. E. C. f. E. a. Health, "Review of evidence on health aspects of air pollution –REVIHAAP Project".

[368]   S. R. Green J, "Perceptions of acne vulgaris in final year medical student written examination answers.".

[369]   Y. B. F. S. Uhlenhake E, "Acne vulgaris and depression: a retrospective examination".

[370]   C. WJ..

[371]   G. J. X. Z. R. L. X. W. Li Wen, "elationship Between Acne and Psychological Burden Evaluatedby ASLEC and HADS Surveys in High School and CollegeStudents From Central China".

[372]   K. H. M.-A. Ismail, "Quality of life inpatients with acne in Erbil city.Health Qual Life Outcomes".

[373]   K. B. K. Y. A. K... A. T. S. D. Yazici, "Disease-specific quality of life is associated withanxiety and depression in patients with acne.".

REFERENCES

[374]   F. D. B. &. V. M. Poli, "An epidemiologicalstudy of acne in female adults: Results o⁻ a survey conducted in France.".

[375]   K. B. M. J. D. A. B. J. K. A. L. Catherine M Nguyen, "The psychosocial impact of acne, vitiligo, and psoriasis: a review".

[376]   G. A. Gupta MA, "Depression and suicidal ideation in dermatology patients with acne, alopecia areata, atopic dermatitis and psoriasis.".

[377]   J. K. U. G. Volker Niemeier, "Acne vulgaris – Psychosomatic aspects".

[378]   https://www.cbsnews.com/news/suicide-pilots-mom-blames-accutane/.

[379]   T. E. S. P. B. J. M. A. Singer S, "Psychiatric Adverse Events in Patients Taking Isotretinoin as Reported in a Food and Drug Administration Database From 1997 to 2017.".

[380]   W. S. Parker Magin, "Isotretinoin, depression and suicide: a review of the evidence".

[381]   https://afsp.org/about-suicide/suicide-statistics/.

[382]   K. W. C. P. B. E. Samad TA, "Regulation of dopaminergic pathways by retinoids: activation of the D2 receptor promoter by members of the retinoic acid receptor-retinoid X receptor family.".

[383]   S. Y. Z. J. e. a. Crandall J, "13-cis-retinoic acid suppresses hippocampal cell division and hippocampal-dependent learning in mice.".

[384]   T. S. B. S. L. M. O'Reilly KC, "13-cis-Retinoic acid alters intracellular serotonin, increases 5-HT1A receptor, and serotonin reuptake transporter levels in vitro.".

[385]   F. N. A. A. V. J. B. M. C. T. V. V. G. M. R. L. S. S. N. C. Bremner JD, "Functional brain imaging alterations in acne patients treated with isotretinoin.".

[386]   S. R. George RM, "Factors Aggravating or Precipitating Acne in Indian Adults: A Hospital-Based Study of 110 Cases.".

[387]   A. H. V. B. Swapna Bondade, "Stressful life events and psychiatric comorbidity in acne–a case control study".

[388]   C. Y. T. S. D. K. H. A. P. G. K. G. Parker G, "Examination stress in Singapore primary school-children: how compliance by subjects can impact on study results.".

[389]   U. EK, "Youth suicide and parasuicide in Singapore.".

[390]   M. T. A. A. G. D. M. C. C. L. G. Y. H. C. a. L. F. S. Gil YOSIPOVITCH, "Study of Psychological Stress, Sebum Production and Acne Vulgaris in Adolescents".

[391]   D. T. A. L. D. E. M. P. S. K. B. Dréno, "Large-scale international study enhances understanding of an emerging acne population: adult females".

[392]   B. T. G. G. P. a. L. E. M.D., "Chronic Stress and the HPA Axis".

[393]   P. D. Mary Ann C. Stephens, "Stress and the HPA Axis".

[394]   H. S. N. H. W. C. M. Y. M. O. W. A. S. C. E. O. S. M. M. S. R. B. Christos C. Zouboulis, "Corticotropin-releasing hormone: An autocrine hormone that promotes lipogenesis in human sebocytes".

[395]   S. A. F. S. G. E. Z. C. Krause K, "Corticotropin-releasing hormone skin signaling is receptor-mediated and is predominant in the sebaceous glands".

[396]   B. C. Melnik, "Acneigenic Stimuli Converge in Phosphoinositol-3 Kinase/Akt/FoxO1 Signal Transduction".

[397]   M. A. S. A. W. J. W. E. M. J. Zbytek B, "Corticotropin-releasing hormone affects cytokine production in human HaCaT keratinocytes".

[398]   E. J. H. a. G. F. Nils Kohn, "Cognitive benefit and cost of acute stress is differentially modulated by individual brain state".

[399]   N. Sousa, "The dynamics of the stress neuromatrix".

[400]   R. M. R. C. M. S. G. Y. W. D. Bandelow B, "Efficacy of treatments for anxiety disorders: a meta-analysis.".

[401]   https://www.camh.ca/en/health-info/mental-illness-and-addiction-index/anti-anxiety-medications-benzodiazepines.

REFERENCES

[402]   "Centers for Disease Control and Prevention (CDC). National Vital Statistics System, Mortality. CDC WONDER Online Database. https://wonder.cdc.gov/. Published 2017. Accessed April 4, 2017.".

[403]   D. A. H. K. D. B. B. L. M. S. Sun EC, "Association between concurrent use of prescription opioids and benzodiazepines and overdose: retrospective analysis.".

[404]   A. J. M. G. V. N. V. A. G. Shiv Gautam, "Clinical Practice Guidelines for the Management of Generalised Anxiety Disorder (GAD) and Panic Disorder (PD)".

[405]   P. B. P. B. P. C. K. K. M. V. A. Martin A Katzman, "Canadian clinical practice guidelines for the management of anxiety, posttraumatic stress and obsessive-compulsive disorders".

[406]   B. M. S. J. B. J. Koszycki D, "Randomized trial of a meditation-based stress reduction program and cognitive behavior therapy in generalized social anxiety disorder.".

[407]   S. V. X. T. A. A. G. C. D. Sofia Tsoli, "Contents lists available atScienceDirectComplementary Therapies in Medicinejournal homepage:www.elsevier.com/locate/ctimA novel cognitive behavioral treatment for patients with chronic insomnia:A pilot experimental study".

[408]   A. M. C. A. M. C. G. C. C. D. Foteini Chatzikonstantinou, "A novel cognitive stress management technique for acnevulgaris: a short report of a pilot experimental study".

[409]   D. D. J. A. W.-P. A. Korabel H, "Psychodermatology: Psychological and psychiatrical aspects of aspects of dermatology.".

[410]   P. A. G. B. C. B. P. T. S. B. ,. V. S. E. M. P. P. D. A. Angelo P., "Recognition of Depressive and Anxiety Disorders in Dermatological Outpatients".

[411]   M. A. N. R. R. K. H. Basavaraj, "Relevance of psychiatry in dermatology: Present concepts".

[412]   https://www.who.int/news-room/fact-sheets/detail/tobacco.

[413]   https://www.who.int/news-room/fact-sheets/detail/tobacco.

[414]   https://www.cdc.gov/tobacco/data_statistics/fact_sheets/health_eff ects/effects_cig_smoking/index.htm.

[415]   "2014 Surgeon General's Report: The Health Consequences of Smoking—50 Years of Progress".

[416]   J. S. M. O. V. B. A. A. M. P. B. Capitanio, "'Smoker's acne': a new clinical entity?".

[417]   S. J. B. V. C. F. P. P. M. Z. C. Capitanio B, "Underestimated clinical features of postadolescent acne.".

[418]   N. A. V. D. B. J. R. J. Schäfer T, "Epidemiology of acne in the general population: the risk of smoking.".

[419]   S. J. O. M. B. V. A. A. P. M. Capitanio B, "Acne and smoking.".

[420]   P. T. F. A. Mills CM, "Does smoking influence acne?".

[421]   K. I. S. T. Z. S. B. S. Klaz I, "Severe acne vulgaris and tobacco smoking in young men.".

[422]   N. T. L. J. Rombouts S, "Cigarette smoking and acne in adolescents: results from a cross-sectional study.".

[423]   M. L. A. J. M. R. B. S. C. C. V. J. T. C. Wolkenstein P, "Smoking and dietary factors associated with moderate-to-severe acne in French adolescents and young adults: results of a survey using a representative sample.".

[424]   M. A. S. J. T. D. V. S. D. A. Wolkenstein P, "Acne prevalence and associations with lifestyle: a cross-sectional online survey of adolescents/young adults in 7 European countries.".

[425]   F. O. L. F. L. T. A. Poli F, "[Acne in adult female patients: A comparative study in France and sub-Saharan Africa].".

[426]   A. J. M. M. M. A. Gonçalves G, "The prevalence of acne among a group of Portuguese medical students.".

[427]   L. A. N. N. F. L. M. F. J. T. Jemec GB, "Have oral contraceptives reduced the prevalence of acne? a population-based study of acne vulgaris, tobacco smoking and oral contraceptives.".

[428]   O. H. Z. C. Ghodsi SZ, "Prevalence, severity, and severity risk factors of acne in high school pupils: a community-based study.".

REFERENCES

[429]   S. R. D. S. N.-K. M. Firooz A, "Acne and smoking: is there a relationship?".

[430]   P. Rev, "Mammalian Nicotinic Acetylcholine Receptors: From Structure to Function".

[431]   J. L. S. M. O. V. B. A. A. M. P. Bruno Capitanio, "Acne and smoking".

[432]   A. C. L. Whitney P Bowe, "Clinical implications of lipid peroxidation in acne vulgaris: old wine in new bottles".

[433]   Y. K. M. I. K. K. O. M. Chiba K, "Comedogenicity of squalene monohydroperoxide in the skin after topical application".

[434]   Y. K. Y. K. M. Egawa, "Oxidative Effects of Cigarette Smoke on the Human Skin".

[435]   D. a. P. W. Church, "Free-radical chemistry of cigarette smoke and its toxicologicalimplications.".

[436]   B. H. J. C. H. W. N. H. G. A. G. S. D. M. Kurzen H, "Phenotypical and molecular profiling of the extraneuronal cholinergic system of the skin.".

[437]   B. D. H. C. G. A. M.-S. N. G. S. K. H. Hana A, "Functional significance of non-neuronal acetylcholine in skin epithelia.".

[438]   B. J. C. A. L. I. Y. X. S. S. H. C. B. S. est KA, "Hana A, Booken D, Henrich C, Gratchev A, Maas-Szabowski N, Goerdt S, Kurzen H.est KA, Brognard J, Clark AS, Linnoila IR, Yang X, Swain SM, Harris C, Belinsky S".

[439]   M. Sopori, "Effects of cigarette smoke on the immune system".

[440]   K. W. S. S. G. Y. K. M. Sopori ML, "Nicotine-induced modulation of T Cell function. Implications for inflammation and infection.".

[441]   https://www.health.harvard.edu/staying-healthy/foods-that-fight-inflammation.

[442]   M. P. H. C. M. P. M. A. S. M. P. a. A. A. M. D. Xiang Gao, "Use of ibuprofen and risk of Parkinson disease".

[443]   P. M. Gagne JJ, "Anti-inflammatory drugs and risk of Parkinson disease".

[444]   S. G. A. G. B.J. Casey, "The adolescent brain".

[445]   G. R. Patterson, "Coercive family process".

[446]   M. S. Bandelow B, "Epidemiology of anxiety disorders in the 21st century".

[447]   "Acne in schoolchildren: no longer a concern for dermatologists".

[448]   A. A. T. C. A. L. N. M. M. P. M. Law, "Acne prevalence and beyond: acne disability and its predictive factors among Chinese late adolescents in Hong Kong".

[449]   G. D. Cunliffe WJ, "Prevalence of facial acne vulgaris in late adolescence and in adults.".

[450]   https://www.insider.com/unique-acne-treatments-2019-5#soaking-your-skin-with-your-own-urine-could-clear-up-your-face-1.

[451]   L. A. J. H. P. a. A. J. Kaspar Sørensen, "Recent Changes in Pubertal Timing in Healthy DanishBoys: Associations with Body Mass Index".

[452]   L. F. E. J. F. F. R. G. F. M. L. L. G. F. W. Sheila F. Friedlander, "Acne Epidemiology and Pathophysiology".

[453]   A. D. I. A. C. J. D. K. &. H. A. Hanson JL, "Cumulative stress in childhood is associated with blunted reward-related brain activity in adulthood".

[454]   N. K. P. A. B. B. Dunn EC, "Is developmental timing of trauma exposure associated with depressive and post-traumatic stress disorder symptoms in adulthood?".

[455]   E. E. W. C. S. C. J. C. K. Mourelatos, "Temporal changes in sebum excretion and propionibacterialcolonization in preadolescent children with and withoutacne".

[456]   M. J. S. S. M. A. D. T. D. P. PETER E. POCHI, "Age-related Changes in Sebaceous Gland Activity".

[457]   R. J. Phillips, "Digital Technology and Institutional Change from the Gilded Age to Modern Times: The Impact of the Telegraph and the Internet".

[458]   H. J. Guyda, "Use of dietary supplements and hormones in adolescents: A cautionary tale".

REFERENCES

[459]   L. R. D., "Insulin-Like Growth Factors".

[460]   "Role of IGF-1 in the Growth Hormone/IGF Axis," [Online]. Available: https://www.alpco.com/role-igf-1-growth-hormoneigf-axis.

[461]   "INSULIN-LIKE GROWTH FACTOR 1(IGF-1) ANDINSULIN-LIKE GROWTH FACTOR BINDING PROTEIN 3(IGFBP-3) GROWTH PANEL".

[462]   J. G. T. C. L. Q. Y. 3. E. J. &. P. P. Imperato-McGinley, "The androgen control of sebum production. Studies of subjects with dihydrotestosterone deficiency and complete androgen insensitivity".

[463]   https://www.britannica.com/science/androgen.

[464]   S. Z. A. C. L. P. C. D. S. F. R. D. R. G. Lombardi *, "Estrogens and health in males".

[465]   R. VA, "Androgens and hair growth".

[466]   S. A. O. C. Z. C. Fimmel S, "Development of efficient transient transfection systems for introducing antisense oligonucleotides into human epithelial skin cells.".

[467]   W. K. Krause, "Plasma DHEA-S levels in adult men and women are 100-500 times higher than those of testosterone and 1000-10000 times higher than those of estradiol".

[468]   G. S. J. I. M. a. K. J. D G Young, "The influence of age and gender on serum dehydroepiandrosterone sulphate (DHEA-S), IL-6, IL-6 soluble receptor (IL-6 sR) and transforming growth factor beta 1 (TGF-β1) levels in normal healthy blood donors".

[469]   L. S. Peter A Torjesen, "Serum Testosterone in Women as Measured by an Automated Immunoassay and a RIA".

[470]   N. C. Usma Iftikhar, "Serum levels of androgens in acne & their role in acne severity".

[471]   M. F. M. B. M. L. A. S. M. J. A. M. P. a. N. W. S. B. Anne W. Lucky, "Predictors of severity of acne vulgaris young adolescent girls: Results of a five-year longitudinal study".

[472]   "What Is a DHEA Test?," [Online]. Available: https://www.webmd.com/healthy-aging/aging-dhea-test.

[473]   M. Anne W. Lucky, M. Frank M. Biro, M. Gertrude A. Huster, A. D. Leach, P. John A. Morrison and R. Joan Ratterman, "Acne Vulgaris in Premenarchal Girls".

[474]   C. M. R. A. B. M. P. M. M. M. P. A. M. J. A. M. C. C. P. S. E. M. L. G. C. O. M. I. G. M. E. D. G. M. M. G. H. G. M. M. D. Alvaro Morales, "Diagnosis and management of testosterone deficiency syndrome in men: clinical practice guideline".

[475]   M. E. L. A. M. a. D. B. M. Tobechi L. Ebede, "Hormonal Treatment of Acne in Women".

[476]   DianeThiboutot1GeorgiannaHarris2VickiIles1GeorgeCimis2KathyrnGil liland1ShinobuHagari, "Diane Thiboutot, Georgiatma Harris, Vicki Iles, George Cimis, Kathyrn Gilliland, and Shinobu Haga".

[477]   H. JB., "Male hormone substance: a prime factor in acne".

[478]   P. P. C. B. K.-P. L. P. L. C. M. C. C. Jiann-Jyh Lai, "The Role of Androgen and Androgen Receptor in the Skin-Related Disorders".

[479]   P. M. E. S. P. A. J. S. .. S. M. DONALD T. DOWNING, "Estimation of Sebum Production Rates in Man by Measurement of the Squalene Content of Skin Biopsies".

[480]   V. P. I. A. R Horton, "Androgen induction of steroid 5 alpha-reductase may be mediated via insulin-like growth factor-I".

[481]   S. L. L. G. T. P. K. a. H. H. Ping Liu, "A Transcription-Independent Function of FOXO1 in Inhibition of Androgen-Independent Activation of the Androgen Receptor in Prostate Cancer Cells".

[482]   I. JT., "Antagonistic effect of androgen on prostatic cell death".

[483]   U. R. C. J. e. a. Ugge H, "Acne in late adolescence and risk of prostate cancer".

[484]   D. J. T. H. H. Yu Zhao, "Modulation of Androgen Receptor by FOXA1 and FOXO1 Factors in Prostate Cancer".

[485]   B. LD., "Acne, its Etiology, Pathology and Treatment.".

[486]   C. V. C. V. A. R. M. I. S. J. Victor Gabriel CLATICI, "Diseases of Civilization – Cancer, Diabetes, Obesity and Acne – the Implication of Milk, IGF-1 and mTORC1".

REFERENCES

[487]   D. FW., "Acne and milk, the diet myth, and beyond.".

[488]   C. A. F. C. Regal P, "Dvelopment of an LC-MS/MS method to quantify sex hormones in bovine milk and influence of pregnancy in their levels".

[489]   A. A. D. S. J. F. H. Frey, "Bioavailability of oral testosterone in males".

[490]   D. S. e. a. Clement A. Adebamowo, "Milk consumption and acne in teenaged boys".

[491]   J. L. J. W. T. K. R Chan, "Associations of dietary protein intake on subsequent decl ne in muscle mass and physical functions over four years in ambulant older Chinese people".

[492]   F. Z. F. S. P. F. V. M. L. C. E. Z. S. T. M. F. Diana Gazzani, "Vegetable but not animal protein intake is associated to a better physical performance: a study on a general population sample of adults".

[493]   Y. O. I. M. D. K. Munehiro Kitada, "The impact of dietary protein intake on longevity and metabolic health".

[494]   https://www.medicalnewstoday.com/articles/323259#high-arginine-foods.

[495]   W. S. B. A. H. M. R. T. Shi L, "Body fat and animal protein intakes are associated with adrenal androgen secretion in children.".

[496]   S. L. B. A. M.-G. C. H. M. W. S. Remer T, "Prepubertal adrenarchal androgens and animal protein intake independently and differentially influence pubertal timing.".

[497]   F. W. L. P. e. a. Ma Q, "FoxO1 mediates PTEN suppression of androgen receptor N- and C-terminal interactions and coactivator recruitment.".

[498]   C. Stringer, "What makes a modern human".

[499]   R. G. Allaby, D. Q. Fuller and T. A. Brown, "The genetic expectations of a protracted model for the origins of domesticated crops".

[500]   Z. MA., "Domestication and early agriculture in the Mediterranean Basin: Origins, diffusion, and impact".

[501]   R. L. McDonald, "The Complete Hamburger: The History of America's Favorite Sandwich".

[502]   E. A. S. D. Zoncu R, "mTOR: from growth signal integration to cancer, diabetes anc ageing.".

[503]   H. H. Lu H, "FOXO1: A potential target for human diseases".

[504]   H.-Z. Z. Moslehi A, "Role of SREBPs in Liver Diseases: A Mini-review".

[505]   "Reference Intervals for Insulin-like Growth Factor-1 (IGF-I) From Birth to Senescence: Results From a Multicenter Study Using a New Automated Chemiluminescence IGF-I Immunoassay Conforming to Recent International Recommendations".